Cancer Biomarkers 3 (2007) 119–121
IOS Press

Foreword

Dean E. Brenner[a] and Gad Rennert[b]
[a]*University of Michigan Medical Center, Ann Arbor, MI 48109-0930, USA*
[b]*CHS National Cancer Control Center, Department of Community Medicine and Epidemiology, Carmel Medical
Center and B. Rappaport Faculty of Medicine, Technion Haifa, Israel*

The six manuscripts in this special issue of Cancer Biomarkers summarize key discussions at the Haifa Prevention Workshop. The workshop, held at the Dan Carmel Hotel in Haifa, Israel from May 4 to May 6, 2004, is an intensive three day meeting that addresses important questions and controversies in translational cancer prevention.

Risk Identification

The issues of environmental exposures and life style were examined by Drs. Leslie Bernstein, Margaret Spitz, Frank Meyskens, Steven Lipkin, Gad Rennert, Paolo Buffeta, Zvi Livneh and Stephen Gruber.

Dr. Bernstein pointed to sufficient data to link col orectal cancer, breast cancer, endometrial cancer, ovarian cancer with exercise and activity. In some of these models, there appears (for example, endometrial cancer) to be a linear relationship with quantity of physical activity and risk of transformation. For colon cancer, job activity correlates with risk of transformation. However, the methodological tools remain problematic. The facets of activity, the time periods, interview reliability of many of the instruments remain problematic. Nevertheless, the link between physical activity and carcinogenesis risk is important and should be developed further through improved data collection instruments.

Dr. Spitz described the increasing linkage between tobacco smoke exposure and genetic function. For example, concordance rates of smoking and nicotine addition are higher among twins than within non-twin families. There is increasing evidence that risk of sustained nicotine dependence is linked to genetic polymorphisms in neurotransmitter systems such as the dopamine pathway, in nicotinic acid receptor structure and function, in metabolic genes (for example, CYP 2A6), and in DNA repair system genes. The current barriers to widespread phenotyping include concerns regarding the specificity of genetic polymorphism functional impact, assay cost and usefulness, incomplete risk assessment models, and weaknesses in biomarker surrogates being used for target tissue endpoint disease.

In the case of melanocyte carcinogenesis, Dr. Meyskens suggested that heavy metal exposure with enhanced oxidation of reactive oxygen species may play a crucial role. Environmental and occupational exposures to redox active metals such as copper, iron, manganese, and lead may enhance carcinogenesis in melanocytes. Chelating agents, environmental modification may be a critical approach to reduction of melanoma.

In the case of colonic carcinogenesis, Dr. Gruber describes in the paper in this issue [1] the large molecular epidemiology study of the I1307K gene missense substitution resulting in a hypermutable tract gives a somatic mutational fingerprint. This haplotype may amplify environmental stress associated with colonic carcinogenesis. For example, in I1307K carriers, vegetable consumption caused at 50% risk reduction in cancer incidence. Physical activity (sports activity) and aspirin or NSAID intake also reduced colon cancer risk.

In a paper published in this issue [2], Dr. Livneh described a new paradigm to risk assessment is being developed through the use of functional assays of critical cellular components that ensure the fidelity of key control systems. DNA repair may be one of these systems. In the case of DNA repair, the cell has multiple pathways to ensure DNA fidelity, some pathways of high quality but with high energy and protein expenditure and others of lower quality but minimal energy expenditure. Polymorphisms in key components of the DNA repair system may impair functionality of these pathways, leading to loss of DNA fidelity in situations of stress. The OGG1 functional assay is one of potentially multiple approaches to interrogate the DNA repair system clinically and provide critical risk assessment information for tumors associated with environmental exposures such as tobacco smoke, lipid peroxidation, and other oxidative stress mechanisms.

The recognition that genetic haplotypes which result in hypermutable genetic segments amplify environmental risk of transformation is a powerful concept that warrants intensive future scientific investigation. Risk assessment in the future is likely to lie with the ability to assess gene environmental interactions functionally. Genetic risk will be based upon haplotype based polymorphic variations that are functionally important. While assessment of genetic risk may be quantified genetically, high throughput, inexpensive functional assays of genetic polymorphisms may be preferable.

Screening and Early Detection

Issues in screening and early detection were addressed by Drs. Sudhir Srivastava, David Ransohoff, Laurence Freedman, Ari Admon, and Robert Bresalier.

Biomarkers should be developed using new high throughput technologies for serious, life threatening illness. Ultimately, biomarkers need some biological plausibility, although one might argue that the products being discovered using high throughput technologies will overwhelm the scientific community's ability to recognize mechanistic linkages. The many barriers to validating biomarkers for the diagnosis or risk assessment of malignant neoplasms have reduced productivity in this field. Among these barriers lead time bias, biosample bias, the gold standards for validation, generalizability, and partially informative markers need to be dealt with systematically for any future success. Among the tools available to minimize the multiple sources of bias are high quality sample ascertainment and storage, training set and test set validation designs, and rigid statistical analysis of variability in both the assay technique and in the diagnostic outcome. Developing and applying these tools requires substantial investment in analytical resources, informatics and biosample repositories, collaborative environments, and skilled personnel.

Dr. Freedman reviewed the statistical issues surrounding the design and analysis of surrogate outcomes [3]. He noted that the aim of interventions is usually to prevent the development of a specific cancer. The most naturally relevant outcome is the occurrence or not of the cancer within a defined long-term time frame; but, long time frames are not feasible with limited resources. Dr. Freedman outlined the different

types of biomarkers surrogates that can be used in place of a cancer occurrence endpoint and suggested that the Prentice model commonly used to determine the dependence of a surrogate upon a specified outcome may not hold for a phase III outcome. Rather, Prentice models should be retained as endpoints in phase II research.

Specific examples of the different approaches to biomarker discovery and validation were addressed by Dr. Srivastava. As described in the paper published in this issue [4], Dr. Admon described the current state of the art and potential future of proteomics. holding great future promise, high throughput proteomics analytics are migrating to a new generation of equipment that will provide better dynamic range and individual protein specificity. The first generation, represented by SELDI, has made important contributions to the concept of high throughput proteome interrogation. Whether this technology will be sufficiently reproducible for clinical applications remains an important research question.

Another example of biomarker development, a mucin glycoprotein product for early detection of colonic malignancy, demonstrates the development of a biomarker through the classical route of mechanism based research identifying a critical product with a role in the carcinogenesis process. This process, while complex and long, results in a discrete product that can be identified using standard analytical methodologies.

Ultimately, success in biomarker based screening and early detection will be based upon the scientific community's ability to integrate diverse analytical tools while maintaining rigorous translational validation in collaborative settings.

Therapeutics

Issues in preventive therapeutics were addressed by Drs. Raju Mehta, Leslie Ford, Nadir Arber, Bernard Levin, Karen Johnson, Powel Brown, Jack Cuzick, Reuben Lotan and Jaak Janssens.

Rodent models remain a crucial preclinical testing tool. Dr. Mehta pointed out that models are developed to describe initiation and promotion schemes. Rodent chemical carcinogenesis models are organ specific and, although not as mechanistically driven as genetically modified models (transgenics, knockouts), remain the mainstay of preclinical efficacy testing because of the ability to model initiation and promotional events. Transgenic models are becoming organ specific and molecular carcinogenesis mechanism targeted. In the future, conditional transgenic models that enable targeted gene and organ site transformation will be important efficacy and biomarker testing models. Chemical carcinogenesis rodent models will remain important in modeling preventive therapeutic efficacy and biomarker responses.

In humans, the movement of preventive therapeutic agents from broad mechanism, such as antioxidant, to targeted agents will continue. Dr. Arber, in his paper published in this issue [5] suggests that cyclooxygenase-2 inhibitors remain important models of targeted agents although recent data suggests that potent targeting of key carcinogenesis associated pathways may have unacceptable toxicity profiles for healthy populations.

Dr. Lipkin notes in his paper published in this issue [6], that existence of multiple regulatory pathway molecules may limit the effectiveness of single targeted agents. Combining targeted agents requires recognition of the complexity of molecular regulation. A "three dimensional" rather than a two dimensional model of activation and inhibitory molecules exists. Targeted therapies may be useful in limited subjects with specific genetic or environmental stresses that have caused deregulation of critical proliferative, apoptotic, and angiogenic regulatory pathways.

The value of large cancer endpoint trials provoked intensive discussion. One advantage of mounting and completing these extensive, expensive trials in addition to identifying efficacy with a cancer endpoint, is the use of these samples an cohorts to ask other important questions. For example, the large tamoxifen breast cancer prevention trial has enable the recognition of tamoxifen's usefulness in BRCA populations, has enabled probing of signal transduction pathways and response to treatment, and has pointed out the need for recognition of dose response clinical pharmacology data.

The development and validation of dietary interventions as opposed to pharmaceutically based interventions was particularly controversial. Diet modulation is the least toxic or expensive preventive intervention available, yet definitive dietary interventions have not prospectively demonstrated efficacy in preventing common cancers. Instruments to quantify diet reproducibly and accurately remain weak. Adherence to diet modulation regimens requires intensive support by professional personnel. Without prohibitively costly professional support, the effectiveness of dietary modulation for cancer preventive efficacy may be limited.

References

[1]   S.B. Gruber, Population Stratification in Epidemiologic Studies of Founder Populations, *Cancer Biomarkers* **3** (2007), 123–128.

[2]   T. Paz-Elizur, D. Elinger, S. Blumenstein, M. Krupsky, E. Schechtman and Z. Livneh, Novel molecular targets for risk identification: DNA repair enzyme activities, *Cancer Biomarkers* **3** (2007), 129–133.

[3]   Laurence Freedman, Quantitative science methods for biomarker validation in chemoprevention trials, *Cancer Biomarkers* **3** (2007), 135–140.

[4]   S.H. Shoshan and A. Admon, Novel technologies for cancer biomarker discovery: Humoral proteomics, *Cancer Biomarkers* **3** (2007), 141–152.

[5]   H. Dvory-Sobol and N. Arber, Cyclooxygenase-2 as Target for Chemopreventive, *Cancer Biomarkers* **3** (2007), 153–161.

[6]   J.L. Velasquez and S.M. Lipkin, Genetic testing to identify high-risk populations for chemoprevention studies, *Cancer Biomarkers* **3** (2007), 163–168.

Cancer Biomarkers 3 (2007) 123–128
IOS Press

Population stratification in epidemiologic studies of founder populations

Stephen B. Gruber*

Departments of Internal Medicine, Epidemiology, and Human Genetics, University of Michigan, Ann Arbor, MI 48109, USA

Abstract. Population stratification represents the principle that genetic variation differs across populations, and these differences may lead to problematic interpretations of epidemiologic studies when the composition of the study population could lead to unmeasured confounding. Advances in genotyping technology greatly facilitate genetic association studies, yet it is critical to understand the relationship between genotype, haplotype, and functional risk alleles. Insights from extended studies of a chromosomal region can provide perspective into the ancestral heritage of founder populations and risk alleles. Examples from studies of colorectal cancer in Ashkenazi Jewish populations, and studies of smoking behavior in Caucasians of European origin, Mexican-Americans, Japanese and Han Chinese illustrate these principles.

1. Introduction

The search for genetic contributions to cancer susceptibility occupies a prominent place in the portfolio of cancer research in the new millennium, and some might argue that this current emphasis is disproportionate to the fraction of cancer that is likely to be attributable to genetic variation. However, fundamental insights into mechanisms of carcinogenesis are emerging in conjunction with successful investigations of genetic variation and cancer, and thus the current commitment to genetic epidemiology seems likely to yield a lush harvest.

The complete draft of the human genome rapidly expanded the possibilities for exploration of genetic variation in epidemiologic studies. In addition, recent studies of the evolution of human populations using data from the HapMap permit investigators to recognize how ancestral patterns of allelic segregation and the structure of human populations are associated with cancer susceptibility [1]. This paper describes some

of the key issues that are relevant to conducting insightful studies that take advantage of both genetic and environmental data.

2. Genotypic variation and risk of cancer

The first studies of cancer susceptibility focused on highly penetrant mutations in cancer genes that could be identified in families with classic Mendelian inheritance such as Familial Adenomatous Polyposis (FAP) and Hereditary Breast Ovarian Cancer Syndrome (HBOC). Early successes in identifying the *APC* gene responsible for FAP and the *BRCA1/BRCA2* genes that cause HBOC led to major advances in clinical care as well as new insights into the pathogenesis of colorectal and breast cancer. Most of the early mutations identified in these genes were easy to interpret, since the functional consequences to the protein were either obvious or simple to predict. However, with further study, subtle genetic variation was recognized that is for more difficult to characterize and understand. Single nucleotide polymorphisms (SNPs) pose a diagnostic challenge, while simultaneously presenting a unique opportunity to understand genetic variation and risk of cancer with a high degree of genomic resolution. SNPs may have direct functional consequences, but they may

---

*Corresponding author: Stephen B. Gruber, MD, PhD, MPH, Division of Molecular Medicine and Genetics, University of Michigan, 4301 MSRB III, Ann Arbor, MI 48109-0638, USA. Tel.: +1 734 615 9712; Fax: +1 734 763 7672; E-mail: sgruber@umich.edu.

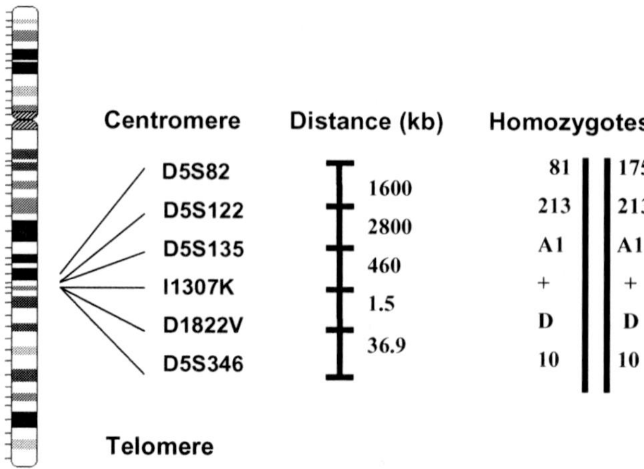

Fig. 1. Haplotype structure of the chromosome 5 region including the APC I1307K susceptibility allele. Microsatellite makers and individual SNPs help distinguish the founder haplotype containing the APC I1307K allele, and genetic distances between markers is useful for estimating the likelihood of recombination events between any two markers. Individuals who carry two copies of the APC I1307K allele illustrate the conservation of a haplotype over reasonably large genetic distances. Note that homozygotes share alleles in the region that extends from D5S122 to D5S346, but that D5S82 is not conserved within this haplotype, Thus D5S82 is outside of the boundary of the conserved allele. Adapted from Niell et al. [3].

also serve as anonymous markers of risk based on the company they keep. In other words, SNPs that are passed along on the same piece of DNA that contains a susceptibility allele for cancer will appear to be associated with cancer due to the close association with the causal mutation rather than the SNPs' inherent properties. As will be discussed below, some SNPs are particularly effective markers of specific configurations of a chromosomal region, and these "haplotype-tagging SNPs" (commonly called htSNPs) can be used to map susceptibility loci.

An example of a SNP with functional consequences that is associated with an increased risk of cancer is the *APC* I1307K polymorphism, found in 6% of Ashkenazi (Eastern European) Jews. First described in an individual with a modest excess of colorectal adenomas, *APC* I1307K confers a two-fold risk of colorectal cancer that accounts for approximately 6% of colorectal cancer in Israel [2]. The polymorphism is a simple missense substitution of isoleucine for lysine in the same gene that is responsible for classic FAP. However, the mechanism of risk seems to be explained by the context of the SNP's surrounding DNA sequence rather than by any recognizable consequence of its predictably inconsequential amino acid substation. Indeed, the SNP is a T>A transversion that creates a repetitive sequence of 8 consecutive adenines, called a polyA tract (A8). Somatic mutational studies show that this polyA tract is particularly vulnerable to DNA replication with imperfect fidelity, and that this DNA sequence serves as a

hypermutable tract where mutations accumulate. Thus APC I1307K is a pre-mutation that confers risk of colorectal cancer as it accumulates subsequent mutations within this hypermutable region of DNA.

SNPs can also reflect inconsequential genetic variation, yet this variation may help provide insight regarding risk conferred by nearby genetic variants. As an example, the *APC* D1822V variant is another reasonable candidate to consider as a potential susceptibility allele. It is a missense polymorphism, and thus one might anticipate that it could have functional consequences. However, bioinformatic predictions suggest that it is more likely to be a neutral polymorphism than one associated with risk of cancer. Indeed, the evidence is overwhelming that D1822V is not directly associated with the risk of cancer in epidemiologic studies, with most studies quantifying the relative risk at about 1.0. This particular polymorphism is located only 1.5 kb from *APC* I1307K, and a recent study shows that almost every individual (98.8%) who carries *APC* I1307K also carriers *APC* D1822V [3]. Therefore, it seems likely that these two SNPs exist on a common ancestral chromosome, which recent studies confirm.

D1822V is far more common than I1307K and is found in a broad diversity of populations. Thus it is not surprising that one can easily separate the risk conferred by I1307K almost exclusively in an Ashkenazi Jewish population from the absence of risk from D1822V. This is possible because D1822V is not found exclusively on ancestral chromosomes that contain I1307K.

of chromosome 5 that have arisen over the history of human evolution, and how these different versions influence the risk of colorectal cancer, one would need to study more than two markers. Indeed, this is the same principle used to take advantage of haplotypes for the genetic association studies.

3. Haplotypes, risk, and genetic anthropology

A haplotype may be defined as a chromosomal region that can be uniquely identified by a small number of genetic markers (such as SNPs or microsatellites) that are embedded within that particular ancestral chromosome. Haplotypes are profoundly useful in increasing the efficiency of genetic association studies, and also provide a window into the complex tapestry of human evolution and ancestral origin. The utility of haplotypes has been greatly facilitated by the HapMap project, an international consortium that has characterized a large fraction of genetic variation within the human genome in different ancestral populations [1,4]. The HapMap project has helped outline the boundaries of extended conserved chromosomal regions that have been preserved through human evolution. These haplotype regions, called blocks, make it possible to use a small subset of markers to identify an entire region of a chromosome that may harbor a susceptibility allele [5]. These conserved haplotype regions also make it relatively straightforward to identify ancestral origin of human populations, so that a reasonably small number of genotypes can distinguish individuals of Asian origin from Africans or Europeans, for example [6–9].

To return to the example of *APC* I1307K, the early recognition that this susceptibility allele was almost exclusively identified in individuals of Ashkenazi Jewish descent suggested that this founder mutation exists on only one ancestral chromosome. Additional genotyping of markers around *APC* I1307K permitted the haplotype to be determined, and the genetic distance of this conserved chromosomal region could be used to calculate the age of the most-recent common ancestor who carried this allele. As shown in Fig. 1, *APC* I1307K does exist on only one version of chromosome 5. The boundaries of this conserved region are related to the likelihood of genetic recombination over time, so a series of calculations make it straightforward to show that *APC* I1307K arose somewhere between 195 BC and 947 BC [3].

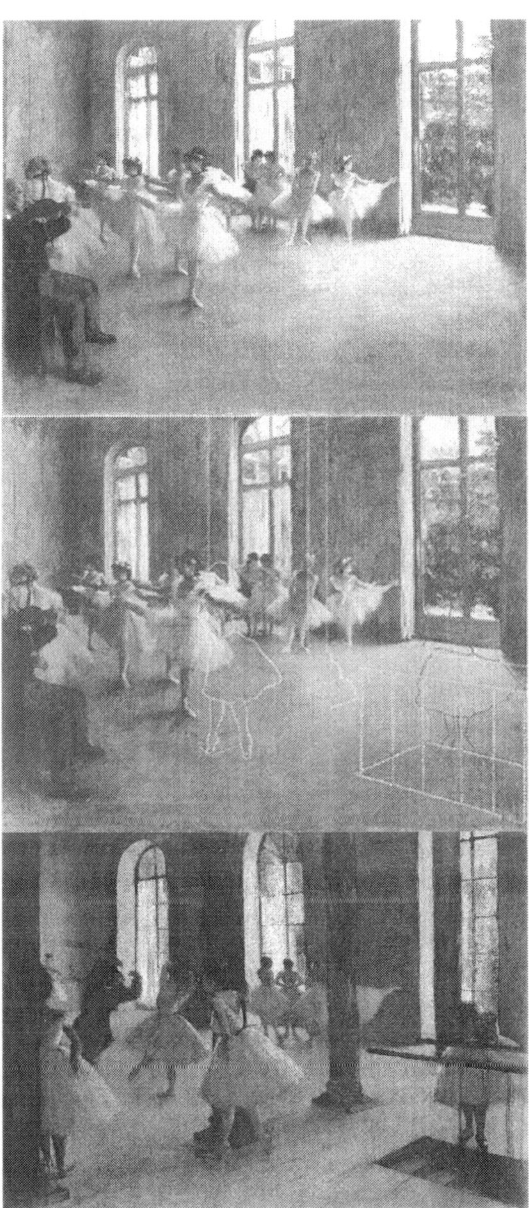

Fig. 2. Principles of population stratification illustrated through a visual analogy. Two paintings of the same population of dancers at a Paris rehearsal hall by Edgar Degas illustrates: a) an open space with a limited number of dancers that can be considered analogous to a founder population, b) radiographic imaging of the same painting shows two other dancers, not visible in the light of the final painting, as well as two columns and a staircase not evident without special consideration of the underlying structure of the painting, and c) a second painting of the same subject, where the light reveals the full extent of the dancer population, as well as the structures supporting the dancers. Courtesy of "Degas and the Dance" [22].

D1822V is readily identified in Jewish and non-Jewish populations, as well as populations of European and African origin. To carefully study the different versions

4. Population structure, unmeasured stratification, and confounding

If a disease is associated with a risk factor that has a different prevalence in one population than in another, then it is important to be account for the differences in the representation of those populations within the study. For example, in a case-control study of smoking and lung cancer, it is possible that smoking rates might differ within different populations at risk, and to accurately measure the risk of lung cancer from smoking within the overall study population one would want to make sure that the case and control groups have similar distributions of subpopulations (eg, Caucasians, African-Americans, Hispanics). Similarly, in studies of genetic risk factors, the possibility that the prevalence of a genetic risk allele might differ within different subpopulations raises the possibility of confounding by population, or what is commonly known as population stratification. Often this type of population stratification is easily recognized by self-report and can be accounted for in the design or analysis of the study. Frequency-matching by race or ethnicity controls for population stratification in the design stage of the study, whereas stratified analysis or logistic regression techniques can account for population stratification within the analysis.

However, sometimes population stratification is not so easily recognized, and other strategies such as genetic cluster analysis is useful to identify cryptic population stratification using unlinked microsatellite markers or SNPs. In populations such as those derived from the US population, ancestral heritage within non-Hispanic Caucasians of European origin is highly unlikely to introduce large biases in epidemiologic studies. Adjustment for cryptic population stratification among non-Hispanic Caucasians of European origin is not always necessary, even though it is technically possible [10, 11]. In other settings, adjustment for cryptic population stratification may be highly advantageous in correctly interpreting an epidemiologic association [12–14]. Spurious associations can arise whenever the allele of interest is differentially represented in one or more populations and when those populations are unequally represented among cases and controls. A specific example offers some perspective about the interpretation of allelic associations in different populations.

5. Haplotypes to the rescue?

The genetic basis of smoking behavior has been investigated in many different populations, and several potentially important candidate genes have been identified. The dopamine D2 receptor (DRD2) is a particularly good candidate since some of the effects of smoking are mediated through dopamine neurotransmission. Epidemiologic studies of smoking probability and intensity have shown that variation in the DRD2 gene is associated with smoking. In Caucasians, both the A1 allele and the nearby B1 allele are associated with smoking probability and intensity. The A1 allele and B1 allele are in a moderately high degree of linkage disequilibrium, as is quantified by the correlation of 0.76 between these alleles. An alternate measure of linkage disequilibrium, D', also shows that these alleles are closely associated, with $D' = 0.464$. Not surprisingly, then, the A1/B1 haplotype is a significant risk haplotype ($p < 0.02$) [15]. In Mexican Americans, the A1 allele is associated with smoking ($p < 0.06$ for linear trend), compared to the A2 allele [16,17]. Therefore, it is rather surprising that the A2 allele (A2/B2 haplotype) is associated with smoking in Japanese men. In fact, the strong association in Japanese men shows that A2/A2 homozygotes are more than twice as likely to be smokers as A1/A1 homozygotes ($OR = 2.32, 95\%$ CI 1.02–5.29) [16,17]. This finding is unlikely to represent a false-positive association, since this Japanese study replicates a prior study demonstrating that the A2 allele is the risk allele among Japanese [18]. What might explain the inverse association between the same allele in different populations?

Even though some have argued that the A1 allele may be a functional polymorphism of the DRD2 gene, recent studies have not been able to demonstrate a significant difference in smoking-induced dopamine release related to the A1 allele by MRI and PET radiotracer imaging [19]. One could hypothesize that the A1 allele is simply a marker allele in linkage disequilibrium with a functional variant that leads to the epidemiologic associations observed in Caucasians and in Mexican-Americans. One could also hypothesize that the opposite allele, A2, is associated with the functional variant in Japanese men.

Data from a fourth population provide additional perspective as well. In the Chinese Han population, the A2/A2 genotype is associated with smoking intensity ($p < 0.047$), consistent with the finding in the two Japanese studies, but in contrast to the studies from North American populations of primarily European descent [20]. This is plausible given current understanding of the genetic anthropology of the Japanese population, since approximately 65% of the gene pool in Japan is derived from continental gene flow from China and Korea around the 3rd century BCE [21].

The true functional variation of DRD2 that may contribute to smoking intensity has not yet been identified, but this example demonstrates the importance of understanding the principles of linkage disequilibrium and population stratification in the interpretation of genetic association studies. Ancestral populations carry the legacy of their gene flow, and genetic variation arising within a specific ancestral context needs to be understood in that context. Genetic associations identified in one population might not be relevant in another population.

As illustrated visually in Fig. 2, the appropriate identification of population stratification in epidemiologic studies requires the appropriate "light". In many circumstances, this "light" can be accomplished with careful questions about ancestral heritage, typically at the level of grandparents. However, sometimes quantitative approaches need to be implemented, which can include methods of genomic control, structured association, principal components, or a new approach using a stratification score, which is the estimated odds of disease calculate using substruture-informative loci data in the disease-odds model [23]. This stratification-score technique has several advantages since it is computationally straightforward, does not assume that the population is composed of discrete subpopulations, and is powerful even in the absence of population stratification.

6. Summary

The principles elucidated here highlight the importance of understanding population stratification in epidemiologic studies. Although the quantitative impact on many studies of relatively homogeneous populations is likely to be trivial, the impact of population stratification in the setting of multiple discrete populations within a study can be profound. This is particularly relevant in studies that include founder populations, since the composition of population structures is often characterized by large disparities in the prevalence of risk alleles. An association between a genetic marker and risk of disease does not necessarily imply that a specific variant is causally linked to the disease, even after adjustment for environmental risk factors. Since it is clear that a genetic variant might be associated with risk of disease purely on the basis of its physical proximity to a causal allele, this type of linkage disequilibrium emphasizes the need to replicate genetic associations in multiple populations as well as to characterize

the functional role of genetic variants. Incorporating these elements into epidemiologic design and analysis protects against spurious associations and facilitates a clearer understanding of the genetic and environmental contributions to disease.

References

[1] A haplotype map of the human genome, *Nature* **437** (2005), 1299–1320.

[2] S.J. Laken, G.M. Petersen, S.B. Gruber, C. Oddoux, H. Ostrer, F.M. Giardiello, S.R. Hamilton, H. Hampel, A. Markowitz, D. Klimstra, S. Jhanwar, S.J. Winawer, K. Offit, M.C. Luce, K.W. Kinzler and B. Vogelstein, Familial colorectal cancer in Ashkenazim due to a hypermutable tract in APC, *Nat Genet* **17** (1997), 79–838.

[3] B.L. Niell, J.C. Long, G. Rennert and S.B. Gruber, Genetic anthropology of the colorectal cancer-susceptibility allele APC I1307K: evidence of genetic drift within the Ashkenazim, *Am J Hum Genet* **73** (2003), 1250–1260.

[4] Integrating ethics and science in the International HapMap Project, *Nat Rev Genet* **5** (2004), 467–475.

[5] L.R. Cardon and G.R. Abecasis, Using haplotype blocks to map human complex trait loci, *Trends Genet* **19** (2003), 135–140.

[6] N.A. Rosenberg, J.K. Pritchard, J.L. Weber, H.M. Cann, K.K. Kidd, L.A. Zhivotovsky and M.W. Feldman, Genetic structure of human populations, *Science* **298** (2002), 2381–2385.

[7] J.K. Pritchard and N.A. Rosenberg, Use of unlinked genetic markers to detect population stratification in association studies, *Am J Hum Genet* **65** (1999), 220–228.

[8] J.K. Pritchard, M. Stephens, N.A. Rosenberg and P. Donnelly, Association mapping in structured populations, *Am J Hum Genet* **67** (2000), 170–181.

[9] D.F. Conrad, M. Jakobsson, G. Coop, X. Wen, J.D. Wall, N.A. Rosenberg and J.K. Pritchard, A worldwide survey of haplotype variation and linkage disequilibrium in the human genome, *Nat Genet* **38** (2006), 1251–1260.

[10] S. Wacholder, N. Rothman and N. Caporaso, Population stratification in epidemiologic studies of common genetic variants and cancer: quantification of bias, *J Natl Cancer Inst* **92** (2000), 1151–1158.

[11] S. Wacholder, N. Rothman and N. Caporaso, Counterpoint: bias from population stratification is not a major threat to the validity of conclusions from epidemiological studies of common polymorphisms and cancer, *Cancer Epidemiol Biomarkers Prev* **11** (2002), 513–520.

[12] D.A. Hinds, R.P. Stokowski, N. Patil, K. Konvicka, D. Kershenobich, D.R. Cox and D.G. Ballinger, Matching strategies for genetic association studies in structured populations, *Am J Hum Genet* **74** (2004), 317–325.

[13] Y. Wang, R. Localio and T.R. Rebbeck, Evaluating bias due to population stratification in case-control association studies of admixed populations, *Genet Epidemiol* **27** (2004), 14–20.

[14] Y. Wang, R. Localio and T.R. Rebbeck, Evaluating bias due to population stratification in epidemiologic studies of gene-gene or gene-environment interactions, *Cancer Epidemiol Biomarkers Prev* **15** (2006), 124–132.

[15] M.R. Spitz, H. Shi, F. Yang, K.S. Hudmon, H. Jiang, R.M. Chamberlain, C.I. Amos, Y. Wan, P. Cinciripini, W.K. Hong and X. Wu, Case-control study of the D2 dopamine receptor

gene and smoking status in lung cancer patients, *J Natl Cancer Inst* **90** (1998), 358–363.

[16] X. Wu, K.S. Hudmon and M.A. Detry, R.M. Chamberlain and M.R. Spitz, D2 dopamine receptor gene polymorphisms among African-Americans and Mexican-Americans: a lung cancer case-control study, *Cancer Epidemiol Biomarkers Prev* **9** (2000), 1021–1026.

[17] N. Hamajima, H. Ito, K. Matsuo, T. Saito, K. Tajima, M. Ando, K. Yoshida and T. Takahashi, Association between smoking habits and dopamine receptor D2 taqI A A2 allele in Japanese males: a confirmatory study, *J Epidemiol* **12** (2002), 297–304.

[18] K. Yoshida, N. Hamajima, K. Kozaki, H. Saito, K. Maeno, T. Sugiura, K. Ookuma and T. Takahashi, Association between the dopamine D2 receptor A2/A2 genotype and smoking behavior in the Japanese, *Cancer Epidemiol Biomarkers Prev* **10** (2001), 403–405.

[19] A.L. Brody, R.E. Olmstead, E.D. London, J. Farahi, J.H. Meyer, P. Grossman, G.S. Lee, J. Huang, E.L. Hahn and M.A. Mandelkern, Smoking-induced ventral striatum dopamine release, *Am J Psychiatry* **161** (2004), 1211–1218.

[20] J. Qi, W. Tan, D. Xing, C. Miao and D. Lin, Study on the association between smoking behavior and dopamine receptor D2 gene polymorphisms among lung cancer cases, *Zhonghua Liu Xing Bing Xue Za Zhi* **23** (2002), 370–373.

[21] S. Horai, K. Murayama, K. Hayasaka, S. Matsubayashi, Y. Hattori, G. Fucharoen, S. Harihara, K.S. Park, K. Omoto and I.H. Pan, mtDNA polymorphism in East Asian Populations, with special reference to the peopling of Japan, *Am J Hum Genet* **59** (1996), 579–590.

[22] J. Devonyar and R. Kendall, Degas and the Dance, *Harry N Abrams* (2002).

[23] M.P. Epstein, A.S. Allen and G.A. Satten, A simple and improved correction for population stratification in case-control studies, *Am J Hum Genet* **80** (2007), 921–930.

Cancer Biomarkers 3 (2007) 129–133
IOS Press

Novel molecular targets for risk identification: DNA repair enzyme activities

Tamar Paz-Elizur[a], Dalia Elinger[a], Sara Blumenstein[a], Meir Krupsky[b], Edna Schechtman[c] and Zvi Livneh[a,*]

[a]*Department of Biological Chemistry, Weizmann Institute of Science, Rehovot 76100, Israel*
[b]*Pulmonary Institute, Sheba Medical Center, Tel Hashomer, Israel*
[c]*Department of Industrial Engineering and Management, Ben Gurion University of the Negev, PO Box 653, Beer Sheva 84105, Israel*

1. Introduction

DNA is continuously damaged by environmental agents and by intracellular byproducts of metabolism [1,2]. If left unrepaired, this DNA damage will cause mutations due to miscoding during replication, thereby increasing cancer risk [1,3]. Therefore, DNA repair is expected to be a major mechanism that protects organisms against cancer. Indeed, in several hereditary diseases that cause high predisposition to cancer, the mutated genes associated with the disorder encode defective DNA repair proteins [3].

2. An overview of DNA repair mechanisms

Over 120 DNA repair genes are known in humans [4], expressing proteins involved in an elaborated system of DNA repair pathways. These pathways can be classified based on their molecular mechanisms and their DNA damage specificity, ranging from highly specific mechanisms directed to a particular type of DNA damage to a DNA repair mechanisms that covers a broad range of DNA damage (see [1] for a comprehensive description). O^6-methylguanine methyl transferase (MGMT; MT) is a protein that specifically demethylates O^6-methylguanine, converting it back to guanine, providing an example of a highly specific reaction performing direct reversal of DNA damage. Base excision repair (BER) is directed to groups of structurally related DNA lesions, and is initiated by one of several DNA glycosylase, which release the modified base from DNA. These includes UDG, that removes uracil from DNA, and OGG1, that removes 8-oxoguanine (8-oxoG) from DNA. The DNA damage specificity of this pathway is determined by the DNA glycosylase, whose action forms in DNA an abasic site. This repair intermediate is repaired by the subsequent action of an abasic site nuclease (termed APE1, HAP1, or APEX), DNA polymerase β and DNA ligase I or III.

Nucleotide excision repair (NER) is a broad range DNA repair process that recognizes a wide variety of DNA lesions, including bulky modifications. It requires multiple proteins, including the products of the seven XPA – XPG genes, the transcription/DNA repair complex TFIIH and other proteins. It involves cuts on both sides of the damage, and release of an oligonucleotide of approximately 30 nucleotides carrying the lesion. The resulting gap is filled in by DNA polymerases δ and/or ε, and sealed by DNA ligase.

Mismatch repair (MMR) corrects replication errors such as base mismatches and small additions or deletions. It acts via excision of a DNA segment carrying the non-matched nucleotide(s), which are recognized

---

*Incumbent of The Maxwell Ellis Professorial Chair in Biomedical Research. Corresponding author: Dr. Zvi Livneh, Dept. of Biological Chemistry, Weizmann Institute of Science, Rehovot 76100, Israel. Tel.: +972 8 934 3203; Fax: +972 8 934 4169; E-mail: zvi.livneh@weizmann.ac.il.

by the MSH2-MSH6 or the MSH2-MSH3 protein heterodimers, and aided by the MLH1-PMS2 or MLH1-MLH3 protein heterodimers. Double strand break (DSB) repair occurs primarily via non-homologous end joining (NHEJ) and involves the proteins Ku, the DNA-dependent protein kinase, the Artemis nuclease and the complex of XRCC4 and DNA ligase IV. DSB repair can occur also by homologous recombination, which involve the RAD51 recombinase, the MRE11-RAD50-NBS1 protein complex, as well as the RAD52 and RAD54 proteins. In addition, there is a tolerance mechanism of translesion DNA synthesis (TLS) that involves replication across DNA lesions that have escaped repair, by low-fidelity specialized DNA polymerases, such as DNA polymerases η, κ, and ζ [1].

3. Reduced DNA repair and the etiology of cancer

The importance of DNA repair mechanisms in cancer etiology is highlighted by several cancer-predisposition hereditary diseases. For example, xeroderma pigmentosum is characterized by sunlight sensitivity and predisposition to skin cancer, and is caused by mutations in genes involved in NER [5–7]. Hereditary non-polyposis colorectal cancer is caused by mutations in mismatch repair DNA genes [8,9]. Mutations in the BER gene MutY, encoding a DNA glycosylase that removes A misincorporated opposite 8-oxoguanine, are associated with MYH-associated polyposis [10], and mutations in the TLS DNA polymerase η cause xeroderma pigmentosum variant, and high predisposition to skin cancer [11,12].

While there is ample evidence for the involvement of DNA repair in hereditary cancer, as described above, the situation in sporadic cancer is less clear. A major reason is the lack of functional specific DNA repair assays that can be used in epidemiological studies. The two DNA assays most frequently used, are the comet assay [13] and the host cell reactivation assay [14]. Using these assays several studies do consistently show that reduced DNA repair is a risk factor in sporadic cancers, e.g., lung cancer [15–17]. However, further insight into the role of DNA repair in the risk of sporadic cancer requires specific functional DNA repair assays that can help elucidate the role of specific DNA repair enzymes or pathways in the development of cancer [18].

4. SNP analysis in DNA repair genes versus functional assays as biomarkers for cancer risk

In recent years there was a large increase in research addressing the role of single nucleotide polymorphisms (SNPs) in DNA repair genes in cancer risk (e.g. [19–21]). The advantages of this approach are impressive: It is simple, fast, high-throughput, and being of germline origin it is relevant to all tissues. However, a particular SNP in a gene is often a poor predictor of the activity of the enzyme encoded by that gene, because it provide only one out of a multitude of factors that affect enzyme activity. These include the methylation status of the gene, transcription, stability of the mRNA, translation, post-translational modification, the presence of inhibitors and stimulators, as well as environmental and lifestyle factors, which are usually very difficult to define. Functional assays are more complex, but they do represent an integrative measure of many of the factors that affect enzyme activity, and are therefore expected to be better predictors of cancer risk [22].

5. The role of the repair of oxidative DNA damage in the risk of lung cancer

The key role of tobacco smoking in lung cancer makes it an attractive system to study the role of DNA repair in sporadic cancer, since tobacco smoke is known to contain 40–50 carcinogens that can cause DNA damage [23,24]. Indeed, several studies have indicated that reduced DNA repair, as assayed by the host cell reactivation assay and the comet assay, is associated with increased cancer risk [15–17]. We decided to develop functional and specific DNA repair assays that can be used for the assessment of lung cancer risk. Our first target was 8-oxoG, a common DNA lesion formed by oxidative stress, ionizing radiation, and tobacco smoke [25]. It may also be incorporated into DNA during DNA synthesis, due to the ability of DNA polymerases to use 8-oxodGTP as a substrate [26]. 8-Oxoguanine is highly mutagenic, causing primarily GC to TA transversions. Remarkably, there are three dedicated mechanisms, conserved from *E. coli* to humans, which act to neutralize the mutagenic activity of 8-oxoG. The main repair mechanism is a sub-pathway of BER, initiated by 8-oxoguanine DNA glycosylase (OGG1), which removes 8-oxoG from DNA. 8-OxoG residues that escaped repair might cause misincorporation of dAMP (instead of the correct dCMP) at a frequency of up to 15%. In these cases a second sub-pathway of BER, initiated by the MYH glycosylase, remove the A, making it possible for a second attempt of DNA synthesis across 8-oxoG to increase the chance of incorporating dCMP, the correct nucleotide opposite 8-oxoG. When this happens, OGG1 can try again to remove the 8-oxoG from DNA (OGG1 acts on 8-oxoG:C pairs, but not on 8-oxoG:A mispairs). The third mechanism that acts to counteract 8-oxoG is via MTH1, an enzyme that specifically hydrolyzes 8-oxodGTP, thereby preventing it from being incorporated into DNA. The fact that these three mechanisms are conserved throughout evolution from *E. coli* to humans indicates it central importance to the maintenance of genomic stability. Moreover, there appear to be several backup mechanisms that can act on 8-oxoG in DNA, including MMR, NER, and NEIL1-initiated BER [1].

We have developed an assay for the activity of OGG, in protein extracts prepared from peripheral blood mononuclear cells [27]. The assay monitors the removal of a site-specific 8-oxoG residue from a synthetic, 32 base pairs-long oligonucleotide. Since OGG activity in the extract causes a break at the site of the lesion, this can be detected after denaturation of the substrate, as a shorter DNA fragment, which can be separated from the uncleaved strand by denaturing polyacrylamide gel electrophoresis.

Using this assay we examined the association of 8-oxoG repair with lung cancer by performing a case-control study with 68 non-small cell lung cancer patients and 68 healthy individuals frequency matched for age and sex. We found that reduced OGG activity is a risk factor in non-small cell lung cancer, with an estimated relative risk (OR) of 4.8 (95% CI 1.5–15.9; $P = 0.01$) for individuals in the lowest tertile of OGG activity compared with individuals in the highest tertile. The adjusted estimated relative risk associated with a unit decrease in OGG activity was 1.9 (95% CI 1.3–2.8; $P < 0.001$). Remarkably, the combination of smoking and low OGG activity caused a greatly increased estimated relative risk for lung cancer. For example, the estimated relative risk of a smoker with a low OGG activity of 4 units/μg protein was 124-fold higher than for a non-smoker with a normal OGG activity of 7 units/μg protein [27]. This high estimated relative risk suggests that the combination of smoking and low OGG activity is responsible for a significant fraction of non-small cell lung cancer cases. If confirmed, this means that screening smokers for low OGG activity may be an effective strategy for lung cancer prevention.

6. Are PBMC an appropriate surrogate tissue for the lung?

The availability of blood specimen makes it the tissue of choice for many epidemiology studies. The question is whether OGG activity measured in PBMC reliably reflects OGG activity in the lung. This is an important issue, since many enzymes, including OGG, exhibit tissue-specific expression. The key point is not the absolute levels of OGG activity, but whether the relative distribution of OGG activity among various tissues is similar in different individuals. In other words, the question is whether if individual A has lower blood OGG activity than individual B, then he/she has a lower OGG activity in the lung (regardless of whether the absolute OGG activities are the same in the lung and in PBMC in the same individual). One way to examine this relationship is by comparing PBMC OGG activity to lung OGG activity whenever the tissue is available. Using such an approach we have found that there was a linear relationship between OGG in PBMC and non-tumor lung tissue from the same individuals, suggesting that an OGG activity in PBMC can serve as a usable surrogate for OGG activity in the lung [27].

7. Does reduced OGG in lung cancer patients represent a risk factor, or is it caused by the tumor?

Like for any other potential risk factor, we first examined whether OGG activity is a risk factor in lung cancer using a case-control study. Indeed, we found reduced OGG activity in non-small cell lung cancer patients compared to healthy subjects frequency matched for age and sex. Such a result can be interpreted by two possible explanations, which have totally different implications: (a) Low OGG is a risk factor in lung cancer. (b) Lung cancer causes a reduction in OGG activity. A case-control study design cannot distinguish between these possibilities, and a definitive answer requires a prospective study. However, in some cases additional experiments can be used to strengthen one of the two possibilities.

In the case of non-small cell lung cancer the main therapy is surgery. Therefore, one can assess the effect of the tumor on PBMC OGG activity by measuring PBMC activity before and after surgery. We measured PBMC OGG activity in non-small cell lung cancer patients from 10 days prior to surgery, up to over one year after the surgery. As can be seen in Fig. 1, OGG activi-

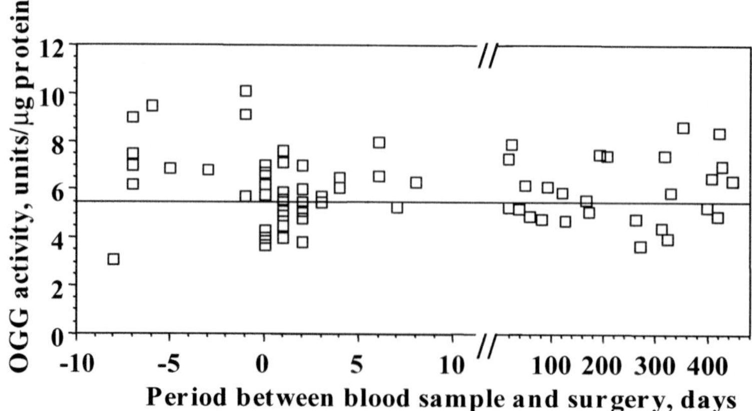

Fig. 1. Effect on OGG DNA repair activity of the time interval between blood drawing and surgery. Blood samples were drawn from 70 non-small cell lung cancer patients at the indicated time periods before or after surgery, and assayed for OGG enzymatic activity.

ties were essentially the same before and after surgery, indicating that the level of OGG activity was not associated with the presence of the tumor. Of course, this is not a definitive proof that the tumor did not cause a decrease in OGG activity, since it is possible that when present, the tumor caused an irreversible decrease in PBMC OGG activity. On the other hand, OGG activity behavior did not change even more than a year after surgery, when at least part of the lymphocyte population was renewed. Taken together these results and considerations, our study suggests that reduced OGG activity is indeed a risk factor in non-small cell lung cancer.

8. DNA repair and target tissue specificity

DNA repair is a housekeeping process, and therefore it is expected to affect all tissue types. However, in practice, DNA repair deficiencies cause tissue-specific clinical symptoms, as seen in the repair-deficiency cancer predisposition syndromes. In those cases, although the DNA repair gene mutation is present in all tissues and cell types, it affects usually one main type of cancer. The reasons for this behavior are not fully understood, but it may involve a situation where there is an excess of the target lesion in a particular tissue. For example, XP patients are defective in NER, the mechanism that repairs most UV- and sunlight-induced DNA damage. Since the skin is the tissue most exposed to sunlight, this may be the reason why XP patients are highly susceptible specifically to skin cancer [7]. Mutations in mismatch repair genes cause primarily colon cancer. In this case, unlike XP, there is no obvious excessive lesion in the colon, and the reason for this manifesta-

tion of cancer-type specificity is not clear. The same behavior might apply to the effect of sub-optimal DNA repair on the risk of sporadic cancer. Thus, reduced OGG activity, shown to be a risk factor in non-small cell lung cancer, is not likely to be a risk factor for all types of cancer, although it might be involved in some cancers other than lung cancer.

9. Future directions

Base excision repair initiated by OGG1 is only one of many DNA repair mechanisms. Therefore, to get a better picture of the role of DNA in cancer risk additional functional DNA repair assays must be developed, and used to assess the contribution of specific repair activities to cancer risk. This must be done for each cancer type separately, since a particular sub-optimal repair activity might affect only a limited number of cancer types, as discussed above. As more DNA repair assays are developed, we might reach a situation in which a battery of DNA repair assays will provide a powerful mean to assess cancer risk in healthy individuals. This may be used to develop effective ways to reduce the incidence of the disease. The case of low OGG activity in smokers can serve as a paradigm for such an approach, because of the large estimated relative risk of 60–200 associated with smokers who have a low OGG activity. The large-scale screening of smokers for low OGG activity might identify individuals at extra-high risk for lung cancer, and those may be more motivated to enter, and successfully complete, smoking cessation programs. Such an approach may lead to a decrease in the incidence of lung cancer.

Acknowledgements

This research was supported by the Associate Members Program of the Early Detection Research Network (EDRN, NCI, NIH, USA), and by the Flight Attendant Medical Research Institute (Florida, USA). Z.L. is the incumbent of the Maxwell Ellis Professorial Chair for Biomedical Research.

References

[1] E.C. Friedberg, G.C. Walker, W. Siede, R.D. Wood, R.A. Schultz and T. Ellenberger, *DNA Repair and Mutagenesis*, (2nd edition), Washington DC: ASM; 2006.

[2] T. Lindahl, Instability and decay of the primary structure of DNA, *Nature* **362** (1993), 709–715.

[3] B. Vogelstein and K.W. Kinzler, *The genetic basis of human cancer*, New York NY: McGraw-Hill; 1998.

[4] R.D. Wood, M. Mitchell, J. Sgouros and T. Lindahl, Human DNA repair genes, *Science* **291** (2001), 1284–1289.

[5] A. Sancar, Mechanisms of DNA repair, *Science* **266** (1994), 1954–1956.

[6] W.L. de Laat, N.G. Jaspers and J.H. Hoeijmakers, Molecular mechanism of nucleotide excision repair, *Genes Dev* **13**(7) (1999), 768–785.

[7] J.E. Cleaver, Common pathways for ultraviolet skin carcinogenesis in the repair and replication defective groups of xeroderma pigmentosum, *J Dermatol Sci* **23**(1) (2000), 1–11.

[8] P. Modrich, Mismatch repair, genetic stability, and cancer, *Science* **266** (1994), 1959–1960.

[9] R.D. Kolodner, Mismatch repair: mechanisms and relationship to cancer susceptibility, *Trends Bioche Sci* **20** (1995), 397–401.

[10] O.M. Sieber, L. Lipton, M. Crabtree, K. Heinimann, P. Fidalgo, R.K. Phillips et al., Multiple colorectal adenomas, classic adenomatous polyposis, and germ-line mutations in MYH, *N Engl J Med* **348**(9) (2003), 791–799.

[11] C. Masutani, R. Kusumoto, A. Yamada, N. Dohmae, M. Yokoi, Yuasa et al., The XPV (xeroderma pigmentosum variant) gene encodes human DNA polymerase eta, *Nature* **399** (1999), 700–704.

[12] R.E. Johnson, C.M. Kondratick, S. Prakash and L. Prakash, hRAD30 mutations in the variant form of xeroderma pigmentosum, *Science* **285** (1999), 263–265.

[13] A.R. Collins, The comet assay. Principles, applications, and limitations, *Methods Mol Biol* **203** (2002), 163–177.

[14] Q. Wei, G.M. Matanoski, E.R. Farmer, M.A. Hedayati and L. Grossman, DNA repair and aging in basal cell carcinoma: a molecular epidemiology study, *Proc Natl Acad Sci USA* **90**(4) (1993), 1614–1618.

[15] Q. Wei, L. Cheng, C.I. Amos, L.-E. Wang, Z. Guo, W.K. Hong et al., Repair of tobacco carcinogen-induced DNA adducts and lung cancer risk: a molecular epidemiologic study, *J Natl Cancer Inst* **92**(21) (2000), 1764–1772.

[16] M.R. Spitz, Q. Wei, Q. Dong, C.I. Amos and X. Wu, Genetic susceptibility to lung cancer: the role of DNA damage and repair, *Cancer Epidemiol Biomarkers Prev* **12**(8) (2003), 689–698.

[17] N. Rajaee-Behbahani, P. Schmezer, A. Risch, W. Rittgen, K.W. Kayser, H. Dienemann et al., Altered DNA repair capacity and bleomycin sensitivity as risk markers for non-small cell lung cancer, *Int J Cancer (Pred Oncol)* **95** (2001), 86–91.

[18] M. Berwick and P. Vineis, Markers of DNA repair and susceptibility to cancer in humans: an epidemiologic review, *J Natl Cancer Inst* **92**(11) (2000), 874–897.

[19] R.J. Hung, J. Hall, P. Brennan and P. Boffetta, Genetic polymorphisms in the base excision repair pathway and cancer risk: a HuGE review, *Am J Epidemiol* **162**(10) (2005), 925–942.

[20] R.J. Hung, P. Brennan, F. Canzian, N. Szeszenia-Dabrowska, D. Zaridze, J. Lissowska et al., Large-scale investigation of base excision repair genetic polymorphisms and lung cancer risk in a multicenter study, *J Natl Cancer Inst* **97**(8) (2005), 567–576.

[21] T. Sakiyama, T. Kohno, S. Mimaki, T. Ohta, N. Yanagitani, T. Sobue et al., Association of amino acid substitution polymorphism in DNA repair genes TP53, POLI, REV1 and LIG4 with lung cancer risk, *Int J Cancer* **114**(5) (2005), 730–737.

[22] T. Paz-Elizur, D.E. Brenner and Z. Livneh, Interrogating DNA repair in cancer risk assessment, *Cancer Epidemiol Biomarkers Prev* **14**(7) (2005), 1585–1587.

[23] S.S. Hecht, Tobacco smoke carcinogens and lung cancer, *J Natl Cancer Inst* **91**(14) (1999), 1194–1210.

[24] J.D. Minna, J.A. Roth and A.F. Gazdar, Focus on lung cancer, *Cancer Cell* **1** (2002), 49–52.

[25] A.P. Grollman and M. Moriya, Mutagenesis by 8-oxoguanine: an enemy within, *Trends Genet* **9** (1993), 246–249.

[26] Y.I. Pavlov, D.T. Minnick, S. Izuta and T.A. Kunkel, DNA replication fidelity with 8-oxodeoxyguanosine triphosphate, *Biochemistry* **33** (1994), 4695–4701.

[27] T. Paz-Elizur, M. Krupsky, S. Blumenstein, D. Elinger, E. Schechtman and Z. Livneh, Reduced DNA repair activity for oxidative damage and the risk of lung cancer, *J Natl Cancer Inst* **95**(17) (2003), 1312–1319.

Cancer Biomarkers 3 (2007) 135–140
IOS Press

135

Quantitative science methods for biomarker validation in chemoprevention trials

Laurence Freedman*
Bar Ilan University and Gertner Institute for Epidemiology and Health Policy Research, Israel

Abstract. Even the most common malignancies have a low probability of occurrence over a restricted time interval. Therefore controlled intervention studies that use incident cancer as an outcome must be large, lengthy and, hence, costly. Studies with surrogate outcomes – biomarkers of pre-clinical carcinogenesis – are attractive because they are potentially smaller, shorter, and less expensive than their counterparts with cancer outcomes.

Despite their potential, however, surrogate outcomes require validation to ensure that they provide sufficient quality of evidence on intervention effects. We review methods that have been proposed over the past 15 years for such validation. The two main approaches are those based on the Prentice criterion, which require data from a single study, and those based on meta-analysis, which require data from many studies. The former approach has fallen out of favor, for reasons to be explained. The latter approach is more popular, but so demanding of resources that it may prove impractical for cancer chemoprevention in all but a few instances. Researchers may have to resign themselves to more limited use of surrogate outcomes, not as replacements for traditional outcomes, but as outcomes for Phase II studies designed to decide which interventions to pass for Phase III testing.

Keywords: Intermediate endpoints, meta-analysis, Phase II chemoprevention studies, Phase III chemoprevention studies, Prentice's criterion, surrogate outcomes, surrogate endpoints

1. Definition and motivation for use of surrogate outcomes

Cancer chemoprevention studies require measures of response to the intervention (outcomes) that are used to judge the value of the intervention strategy. Since the aim of the intervention is usually to prevent the development of a specific cancer, the most naturally relevant outcome is the occurrence or not of the cancer within a defined long-term time frame. A serious problem faced by researchers in cancer prevention is that such outcome measures necessitate studies with large numbers of individuals (because of the rarity of most cancers) observed over long periods of time [1]. These studies are very expensive and obtaining funding for them is notoriously difficult.

For this reason researchers have searched for alternative designs. One of these is the substitution of alternative shorter term outcomes in place of cancer development. These alternative outcomes have been called *surrogates, surrogate endpoints* or *surrogate outcomes*. In the context of cancer chemoprevention such surrogates are usually biomarkers, measures of genetic, biochemical, cellular or tissue processes that are in some way connected to the cancer (see below).

There has been some confusion of the exact definition of a surrogate outcome. A simple definition is any measure of intervention response that can be made between the initiation of the intervention and the development of cancer, with the intention of using it in place of the cancer outcome. Although some would view this definition as being too wide because it potentially includes measures that are so weakly linked to cancer development as to be of no practical use, I adopt this definition in this article.

At the other end of the scale of specificity, a very strict definition of a surrogate outcome is one that *lies*

*Present address: Biostatistics Unit, Gertner Institute for Epidemiology and Health Policy Research, Tel Hashomer 52161, Israel. Tel.: +972 3 5305390; E-mail: lsf@actcom.co.il.

on the causal pathway between the intervention and the cancer. While the causal pathway property is clearly very desirable for a surrogate outcome, some view this definition as operationally unhelpful as it is often exceedingly difficult to demonstrate causality in medicine. However, it is useful to distinguish outcomes for which we are able to infer with a fair amount of certainty that this conditional holds. Therefore I will call such outcomes *"causal"* surrogates although this is not a term that has been used in the literature.

I have already mentioned that a major motivation for identifying a surrogate outcome is the aim of shortening and reducing the cost of clinical trials of cancer prevention. However, deeper motivations for identifying a causal surrogate are the understanding of the etiology of the cancer and, ultimately, devising new methods of prevention. An example is the identification of Human Papillomavirus (HPV) as a (probably causative) risk factor for cervical cancer [2]. HPV infection is now used as a surrogate outcome in some cancer prevention trials, but more importantly it suggests a new way of preventing cancer of the cervix through HPV vaccination [3].

In this article I will review the difficult questions of what makes a good surrogate outcome, how one might validate a surrogate outcome, and whether the approaches to validation proposed in the literature are likely to be of benefit to the design of cancer chemoprevention studies. Before embarking on this we need to consider what surrogate outcomes might be used in cancer prevention studies.

2. Surrogates for the cancer outcome

Clearly a surrogate needs to be related to the cancer process in some way. There is, of course, a wealth of information on factors that are thought to be related to cancer, although the level and clarity of the underlying evidence varies enormously from factor to factor.

There are four main classes of biomarkers that may be considered as possible surrogates for cancer outcomes [4].

2.1. Alterations in tissue characteristics

Examples include cervical intraepithelial neoplasia (CIN), prostatic intraepithelial neoplasia (PIN), colonic adenomatous polyps,and mammographic parenchymal patterns. Usually such alterations occur quite late in the carcinogenic process and one may therefore expect the

relationships with the cancer outcome to be stronger. However not all CINs or adenomatous polyps proceed to cancer, so the relationship is far from a perfect one. In addition, the further the alteration occurs in time along the cancer pathway, the longer time one may need to wait to observe the effect of the intervention. See the end of Section 4.1 for further discussion.

2.2. Cellular phenomena

Examples include cell proliferation markers and apoptosis markers. These are markers that may be more rapidly influenced by interventions than are tissues, but whose relationship to the cancer outcome is more distant and therefore generally weaker.

2.3. Molecular markers

Examples include somatic mutations (RAS, TP53), DNA hypo- and hyper-methylation of specific genes, and gene-expression products.

2.4. Infection and inflammation

Examples include HPV, Helicobacter pylori, inflammatory cells, and cytokines.

3. What is a good surrogate?

The answer to this question has to be related to how we intend to use the surrogate. Since the discussion here relates to using surrogates in place of cancer outcomes in a cancer prevention trial, the answer has to be that a good surrogate is one that predicts well the effect of the intervention upon the cancer outcome.

Note that this pragmatic answer allows for the possibility that a biomarker may be a good surrogate for cancer outcome for one intervention but not for another. To give a very simple example, in preventing lung cancer, smoking prevalence may be a very good surrogate for cancer outcome in a trial of a smoking cessation program, but is clearly of no use in a trial of an antioxidant.

The above example also illustrates that a causal surrogate (cigarette smoking for lung cancer) is not necessarily a good surrogate (as in the antioxidant trial). Nevertheless being on the causal pathway to the cancer is obviously a desirable property for a surrogate outcome that will often enhance its predictive ability.

Table 1
Number of sexual partners and the risk of cervical dysplasia (taken from Schiffman et al. [2])

	Number of sexual partners				
Odds Ratio	1	2	3–5	6–9	10+
Unadjusted	1.0	1.7	3.1*	4.7*	4.4*
Adjusted for HPV	1.0	1.0	1.1	1.5	1.6

$*P < 0.05$.
HPV Human Papilloma Virus Infection.

We now turn to the questions of judging how well a surrogate outcome predicts the effect of intervention on the cancer outcome, and obtaining some operational approaches to this evaluation. This topic has come to be known in the biostatistical literature as "surrogate outcome validation".

4. Approaches to validation

Two main approaches to validation have been taken, namely model-based and empirical. We examine each in turn.

4.1. Model-based approaches

The first statistically oriented approach to validation was that taken by Prentice [5]. The model on which the method is based may be illustrated graphically, as in Fig. 1, part (a). Intervention or exposure (E) affects surrogate (S) which in turn affects cancer outcome (T) [6]. This idealized model means that the entire effect of exposure or intervention on cancer outcome is mediated through the surrogate, and is the ideal situation for the use of a surrogate in a trial of the intervention (or in an epidemiologic study of the exposure). Of course, there may be other pathways to the cancer outcome, but as long as they act completely independent of the E-S-T pathway illustrated then the situation remains ideal for the surrogate. Prentice's approach cannot be described technically without using statistical theory, but the main idea is that the "Prentice criterion" holds when this ideal situation exists.

A simple alternative model is shown in Fig. 1, part (b), where the intervention or exposure affects both the surrogate S and a second independent pathway to cancer, measured by M. In this case the Prentice criterion no longer holds [6].

Although enunciating this criterion was a big step forwards in conceptualizing the idea of a "valid" surrogate, its application has been difficult. Firstly, in regard to cancer outcomes, biologists believe that the situa-

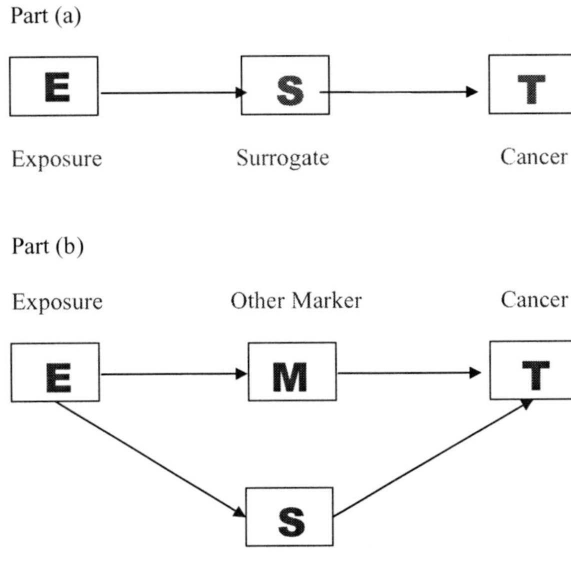

Fig. 1. Idealized schema illustrating possible relationships between exposure (E), surrogate (S) and cancer outcome (T).

tions in which the Prentice criterion would hold must be very rare. Secondly, even when such situations may exist, it turns out to be extremely difficult operationally to verify that the criterion holds.

Freedman et al. [7] pointed out that a validation analysis attempting to verify that the Prentice criterion holds for a certain surrogate can be conducted using data from a randomized clinical trial that includes assessment of both the cancer outcome and the surrogate in each individual. First we estimate the intervention effect on the cancer outcome and hope that it is significantly different from zero (preferably at a high degree of statistical significance). If it is not statistically different from zero then we can make no progress in the validation analysis. Suppose that we next estimate the intervention effect adjusted for the surrogate. If the adjusted effect disappears (becomes zero) then Prentice's criterion holds.

Two examples will illustrate the idea. The first example relates to the epidemiology of cervix cancer. The exposure is the number of sexual partners, the surrogate is HPV infection and the outcome is cancer of the cervix. Table 1 displays data from a case-control study reported by Schiffman et al. [2]. The unadjusted relative risk for cervix cancer from 6–9 or more than 10 partners is estimated to be above 4, in keeping with many other epidemiologic studies of risk factors for this cancer. Adjustment for HPV infection reduces the estimated RR to 1.5–1.6. The reduction is dramatic although the effect after adjustment does not disappear completely, as required to declare that the Prentice criterion holds. Nevertheless this impressive result clearly leaves the impression that HPV explains nearly if not all of the association between number of sexual partners and cervix cancer, which would indicate the near validity of using HPV as a surrogate for cancer in other studies relating sexual activity to cervix cancer.

The second example concerns a cholesterol lowering drug and its effect on heart disease. In the randomized LRC trial of cholestyramine in 3806 males with hypercholesterolemia (Ref), the percentage of myocardial infarctions (MI) or CHD deaths in the placebo group was 8.8% compared to 6.9% in the cholestyramine group. In a logistic regression model the log odds ratio for MI/CHD death from cholestyramine was -0.26 (approximately a reduction of 26%) with a standard error of 0.12. After adjustment for the cholesterol level after 1 year of treatment, the adjusted log odds ratio was -0.13 (approximately a 13% reduction) with a standard error of 0.13 [7]. The reduction is modest, with the adjusted estimate about half of the unadjusted. Moreover, the 95% confidence limits for the adjusted estimate indicates that the true adjusted effect could be as low as -0.13 or as high as 0.39, encompassing both the case where the Prentice criterion holds (0) and the case where the surrogate plays no mediation role in the relation between cholestyramine and heart disease (0.26). Thus the result of the analysis is essentially uninformative.

The first example is one of the rare successes of the Prentice criterion approach in cancer etiology research. Unfortunately, the second example is more typical of the results that are usually obtained. The barriers to success for this approach include the following.

(a) One usually cannot estimate the adjusted effect with sufficient precision to know when it's truly equal (or close) to zero;

(b) Sufficient precision is usually possible only when the unadjusted effects are very highly significant (with z-values of 3.5 or above); such effects are rarely observed in clinical trials, particularly in the era of data and safety monitoring when clinical trials are terminated before such levels of significance are reached. The method holds more promise in epidemiological settings where highly significant unadjusted effects are more commonly found.

(c) Even when a surrogate has been successfully validated using this method, the validation is good only for the intervention or exposure used in the study. The surrogate may not necessarily be used safely for a study involving a different intervention.

After a volley of papers criticizing this approach [8–11], the method is now out of favor, at least for clinical trials applications.

A different, indirect, approach to establishing that the Prentice criterion holds is via the attributable risk (AR) of the surrogate. The AR is an estimate of the proportion of cases of the cancer that can be attributed to a given risk factor [12]. If this is sufficiently high (say over 90%), then the pathway through S in Fig. 1 is the only important one and the conditions of Fig. 1, part (a) will therefore hold approximately. Thus biomarkers with very high AR's may be excellent surrogates. The estimate of the AR for HPV is now over 0.99 [13]. Adenomatous polyps are thought to account for over 90% of colon carcinomas that develop [14], and have been used as surrogates in cancer chemoprevention trials [15,16]. Once again, situations in which such high AR's are found are unfortunately rare.

Even in the case where a surrogate has a high AR, inferences that can be made from a trial using the surrogate as the outcome are not straightforward. For the problems in making inferences about cancer from trials of adenomatous polyp occurrence see Schatzkin et al. [14].

4.2. Empirical approaches

Whereas the model-based approaches to validation described above require data on a single study only, the empirical approaches rely on a meta-analysis of many studies. One of the earliest examples of this approach is described by Daniels and Hughes [17], who analyze 24 treatment comparisons from randomized trials of treatments for AIDS. A summary of their data is shown in Fig. 2, which displays a plot of the estimated effect of treatment on clinical outcome (the log hazard ratio) against the estimated effect of treatment on the surrogate (the change in CD4 cell count).

The main idea behind the empirical approach is to establish a relationship between the effects on the clinical outcome (T) and the surrogate (S), and then to use this relationship to predict the effect on T in a new study that is designed to estimate only the effect on S. Naturally, great care must be placed on placing confidence limits around the prediction. When the relationship seen in the meta-analysis is a fairly weak one, then the prediction will be more uncertain and the confidence

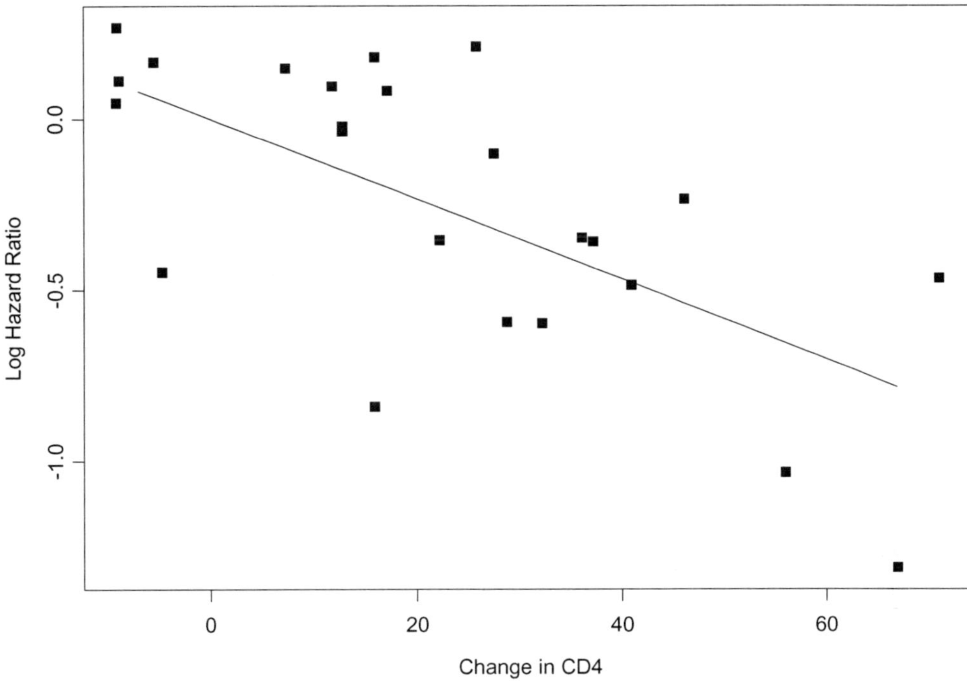

Fig. 2. Plot of estimated effects of treatment on survival versus change in CD4 count for 24 treatment comparisons (taken form Daniels and Hughes [17]).

limits will be wide. Different versions of this approach have been described by Daniels and Hughes [17], Gail et al. [18], Molenberghs et al. [19] and Korn et al. [20] among others. A book summarizing this work has recently been published [21].

These methods have several advantages over the model-based approach. First, they are driven by past experience over a series of studies, and in that sense are less speculative than those based on an idealized model of the intervention-surrogate-cancer outcome relationship. Second, the meta-analysis can incorporate different treatments, so that the validation is usually less heavily based on a single treatment than is the model-based approach. Third, unlike the Prentice criterion approach, the meta-analysis can include trials for which non-significant estimates of treatment effect are obtained.

Nevertheless, there are also several limitations to the approach. The most serious of these is the data required of the method. For successful application, there must be available data from many studies, each of which includes measurements of the same surrogate and the same cancer outcome. Moreover, these studies must be of reasonable size, so that the estimates of treatment effects on the cancer outcome and on the surrogate are reasonably precise. Attempts to increase

the number of studies artificially by dividing a single multi-center study into several single-center studies are unsuccessful because each treatment effect is estimated very imprecisely.

5. Discussion

Cancer chemoprevention trials with cancer outcomes are very time-consuming and expensive undertakings. If we could discover a way of evaluating reliably a chemopreventive agent through use of a surrogate outcome instead of the cancer outcome, this would be an important contribution to the field. However, the methods described in this paper do not appear very promising approaches to validating surrogates for chemoprevention trials.

The Prentice criterion approach has not been found helpful when used on data from randomized trials and has fallen from favor. The attributable risk approach works only for the rare surrogates that have very high AR's. The empirical approaches require data that are not usually available in the cancer chemoprevention context. The number of randomized clinical trials of chemoprevention with a cancer outcome that have been performed over the past 15 years is relatively small, and when one divides these into cancer type and surrogate biomarker of interest they will rarely amount to more than two per case. Thus there seems little or no database on which to conduct this approach.

We may therefore ask whether biomarkers will be of any use in evaluating cancer chemoprevention agents, and if so how? I believe the role for biomarkers is not at the stage of definitive (Phase III) evaluation of an agent, but in identifying promising agents at the Phase II stage of evaluation. The choice of which biomarkers to use should be based on the known or hypothesized biological mechanism of the agent. Clearly, if the relationship of that biomarker to the cancer outcome is strong then the evidence for moving the agent into Phase III trials will be correspondingly stronger. However, it seems wise to allow a range of designs of Phase II studies, some with biomarkers that are closer to the intervention (closer to markers of exposure than markers of cancer) that one might call "early" Phase II, and some with biomarkers somewhat closer to the cancer outcome that one might call "late" Phase II studies.

Acknowledgments

The author acknowledges Arthur Schatzkin, Mitchell Gail and Mark Schiffman of the US National Cancer Institute for previous collaboration and many valuable discussions on these issues.

References

[1]   D.P. Byar, The design of cancer prevention trials, *Recent Results Cancer Res* **111** (1988), 95–98.

[2]   M.H. Schiffman, H.M. Bauer, R.N. Hoover, A.G. Glass, D.M. Cadell, B.B. Rush et al., Epidemiologic evidence showing that human papillomavirus infection causes most cervical intraepithelial neoplasia, *J Natl Cancer Inst* **85** (1993), 958–964.

[3]   J. MacLean, E.P. Rybicki and A.L. Williamson, Vaccination strategies for the prevention of cervical cancer, *Expert Rev Anticancer Ther* **5** (2005), 97–107.

[4]   A. Schatzkin and M. Gail, The promise and peril of surrogate end points in cancer research, *Nat Rev Cancer* **2** (2002), 19–27.

[5]   R.L. Prentice, Surrogate endpoints in clinical trials: definition and operational criteria, *Stat Med* **8** (1989), 431–440.

[6]   A. Schatzkin, L.S. Freedman, M.H. Schiffman and S.M. Dawsey, Validation of intermediate end points in cancer research, *J Natl Cancer Inst* **82** (1990), 1746–1752.

[7]   L.S. Freedman, B.I. Graubard and A. Schatzkin, Statistical validation of intermediate endpoints for chronic diseases, *Stat Med* **11** (1992), 167–178.

[8]   M. Buyse and G. Molenberghs, Criteria for the validation of surrogate endpoints, *Biometrics* **54** (1998), 1014–1029.

[9]   P.W. Bycott and J.M. Taylor, An evaluation of a measure of the proportion of the treatment effect explained by a surrogate marker, *Control Clin Trials* **19** (1998), 555–568.

[10] P. Flandre and Y. Saidi, Estimating the proportion of treatment effect explained by a surrogate marker, *Stat Med* **18** (1999), 107–109.

[11] G. Molenberghs, M. Buyse, H. Geys, D. Renard, T. Burzykowski and A. Alonso, Statistical challenges in the evaluation of surrogate endpoints in randomized trials, *Control Clin Trials* **23** (2002), 607–625.

[12] J. Benichou, Attributable Risk, in: *Encyclopedia of Biostatistics*, 2nd, P. Armitage and T. Colton, eds, edition, Wiley, Chichester, UK, pp. 249–262.

[13] J.M. Walboomers, M.V. Jacobs, M.M. Manos, F.X. Bosch, J.A. Kummer, K.V. Shah et al., Human papillomavirus is a necessary cause of invasive cervical cancer worldwide, *J Pathol* **189** (1999), 12–19.

[14] A. Schatzkin, L.S. Freedman, S.M. Dawasey and E. Lanza, Interpreting precursor studies: what polyp trials tell us about large-bowel cancer, *J Natl Cancer Inst* **86** (1994), 1053–1057.

[15] J.A. Baron, M. Beach, J.S. Mandel, R.U. Van Stolk, R.W. Haile, R.S. Sandler, R. Rothstein, R.W. Summers, D.C. Snover, G.J. Beck, J.H. Bond and E.R. Greenberg, Calcium supplements for the prevention of colorectal adenomas. Calcium Polyp Prevention Study Group, *N Engl J Med* **340** (1999), 101–107.

[16] A. Schatzkin, E. Lanza, L.S. Freedman, J. Tangrea, M.R. Cooper, J.R. Marshall, P.A. Murphy, J.V. Selby, M. Shike, R.R. Schade, R.W. Burt, J.W. Kikendall and J. Cahill, The polyp prevention trial I: rationale, design, recruitment, and baseline participant characteristics, *Cancer Epidemiol Biomarkers Prev* **5** (1996), 375–383.

[17] M.J. Daniels and M.D. Hughes, Meta-analysis for the evaluation of potential surrogate markers, *Stat Med* **16** (1997), 1965–1982.

[18] M.H. Gail, R. Pfeffer, H. Van Houwelingen and R.J. Carroll, On meta-analytic assessment of surrogate outcomes, *Biostatistics* **1** (2000), 231–246.

[19] G. Molenberghs, H. Geys and M. Buyse, Evaluation of surrogate endpoints in randomized experiments with mixed discrete and continuous outcomes, *Stat Med* **20** (2001), 3023–3038.

[20] E.L. Korn, P.S. Alberts and L.M. McShane, Assessing surrogates as trial endpoints using mixed models, *Stat Med* **24** (2005), 163–182.

[21] T. Burzykowski, G. Molenberghs and M. Buyse, eds, *The Evaluation of Surrogate Endpoints*, Springer Verlag, New York, 2005.

Cancer Biomarkers 3 (2007) 141–152
IOS Press

Novel technologies for cancer biomarker discovery: Humoral proteomics

Stacy H. Shoshan and Arie Admon*
Department of Biology, Technion-Israel Institute of Technology, Haifa 32000, Israel

Abstract. The repertoires of serum autoantibodies differ between healthy people and cancer patients. While in healthy individuals these autoantibodies are directed against a limited number of self-proteins, in cancer patients the antibody repertoires are much further expanded with a wider range of reactivities against other proteins. Although cancer patients clearly mount humoral immune responses, they are not very effective in preventing the progression of the disease. However, the implication from the presence of these new and abnormal antibody specificities relates to their potential as novel tools for early detection before clinical manifestations. Proteomics technologies, with their unique ability to identify both tumor antigens and their cognate serum autoantibodies, hold great promise in facilitating the development of early detection kits and possibly also as conduits for the isolation of tumor antigens for immunotherapy.

Keywords: Humoral proteomics, serological proteomics, SEREX, autoantibodies, mass spectroscopy, 2D-electrophoresis, protein arrays

1. Humoral proteomics terminology

While many laboratory groups are combining proteomics with serological analysis to identify tumor antigens and serum autoantibodies, the different methodologies are being called by unique names. For example, there is SERPA [1], SPEAR [2], PROTEOMEX [3], and Ab SCAN [4]. To further the problem of confusing terminology, many groups refer to examining the serum proteome as serological proteomics [5]. Therefore, we propose that the term humoral proteomics be exclusively and inclusively used to define research involving proteomics techniques that strive to identify both target antigens and serum autoantibodies. This would greatly facilitate connections and ease the literature search, and possibly avoid further ambiguity associated with the term serological proteomics.

2. Conventional proteomics technologies

The main technologies of any proteomics study are two-dimensional polyacrylamide gel electrophoresis 2D-PAGE [6], capillary high-performance liquid chromatography (μHPLC), and mass spectrometry (MS) (reviewed in [7]). First, target populations of cancer cells need to be isolated from tissue sections in the operating room, biopsy samples, cultured cell lines, or serum. Proteins are then extracted from the cancer cells and separated using 2D-PAGE or HPLC. One of the major advances in 2D-PAGE technology was the replacement of classical first-dimension carrier ampholyte pH gradients with well-defined immobilized pH gradients [8]. This innovation alone has resulted not only in higher resolution, but most importantly in more easily reproducible gels. Unfortunately, 2D-PAGE is not an automated technique, thus making it operator-dependent, time-consuming, and labor-intensive. It requires a relatively large amount of protein as starting material, and it is limited in its ability to handle proteins that are very large, very small, basic or hydrophobic. Visualization methods for protein detection within the gels vary in their limits of detection and dynamic range.

*Corresponding author: Arie Admon, Tel.: +972 48293407; Fax: +972 48225153; E-mail: admon@tx.technion. ac.il.

Compatibility with MS analysis includes staining with Coomassie, sliver, zinc-imidazole and several types of fluorescent dyes (reviewed in [9,10]).

When 2D-PAGE is used, multiple gels are usually run together, so that one can be stained while the others are used for western blotting. The western blots are probed with serum of cancer patients or control donors to search for antigens that exclusively react with the antibodies of the cancer. Serum used for comparison as a control can be from healthy people, individuals with tumors other than the target cancer, or patients with other diseases. Protein spots from the western blots that are solely reactive with antibodies from cancer serum can then be excised from the corresponding stained gels for identification by standard proteomics technologies and further study. These proteins of interest are *in-gel* digested, analyzed using tandem mass spectroscopy (MS/MS), and then identified using bioinformatics tools.

An alternative protein separation technique is HPLC. One-, two- and multidimensional HPLC is a viable preparatory step for isolating tumor antigen repertoires, which can be followed by printing the resolved proteins on proteins arrays for probing with serum antibodies. Two-dimensional HPLC is often used, where the first dimension separation is strong cation exchange, and the second reversed-phase. HPLC, unlike 2D-PAGE, can be fully automated and interfaced directly to MS. The main drawback of HPLC is the low recovery rate of some proteins that "stick" to the columns.

MS can be used to identify proteins with only minute amounts of material (reviewed [7]). MS is currently the optimal technology for studying posttranslational modifications (PTMs) which affect protein function, activity, stability, localization and turnover (reviewed in [11,12]). Tumor cells often have aberrant proteins that differ from their wildtype counterparts, sometimes only in having PTMs or expression as different isoforms. MS is often the only technology capable of detecting these variances. Furthermore, MS technology has become increasingly automated and more easily interfaced to bioinformatics tools. For example, "spot-picking robots" can transfer protein spots from 2D-PAGE gels to microtitre plates, which then undergo a completely automated regimen. The proteins are processed unstained and trypsin-digested with the resulting peptides analyzed and identified using MS/MS. This level of efficiency allows for up to thousands of protein spots per day to be analyzed [13]. Based on the MS-generated peptide sequences, dedicated software tools are then used to facilitate identification of proteins and their encoding genes.

Protein, antibody and tissue arrays are at the forefront of the new era of large-scale, high-throughput proteomics technology. They present a rapid and economically feasible tool that could represent the future of proteomics early detection kits. While protein arrays are based on the successful model of DNA arrays, proteins are more complex molecules than nucleic acids and therefore are more challenging to configure into arrays. Proper interactions with other molecules, such as antibodies, often require that the antigenic portion be retained in its native conformation even after treatment with buffers or other reagents used for protein extraction.

All arrays are based on the same principle, namely, an immobilized molecule, such as a protein, is probed by a tagged molecule, like a protein or an antibody from serum or cell lysates (reviewed in [14]). Functional arrays are used to assay for biochemical activity, whereas analytic arrays are used to detect proteins in a complex mixture (reviewed in [15]). Analytic arrays can be used to generate patterns of binding reflecting temporal changes in protein repertoires of tumor antigens and autoantibodies such as in diseased/non-diseased states and before/after treatments. Hanash and his colleagues developed a protein microarray based on A549 lung adenocarcinoma cell lysates. They used a two-dimensional HPLC protein fractionation system to separate the intact proteins that contained their native PTMs, and then spotted them onto microarrays which were probed with serum from newly diagnosed patients with lung cancer and healthy controls. They were able to identify a series of tumor antigens that induced an antibody response in the cancer patients, which resulted in a reproducible pattern of reactivity [16].

The Hanash group used the 2D-HPLC also to separate proteins from the prostate cancer cell line LNCaP into fractions that could be spotted onto microarryas. They investigated whether certain fractions exhibit antibody binding and whether the serum from the prostate cancer patients could be classified based on its patterns of humoral immune reactivity. A decision tree with two levels of partitioning classified serum samples from 25 men with prostate cancer and 25 male controls with 98% accuracy (1 misclassification). Their results demonstrate the possibility that using microarrays of fractionated proteins, patterns of immune recognition can be used as diagnostic tests by measuring serum antibody reactivities to multiple prostate cancer antigens [17].

3. Autoantibodies: Friend, foe or mysterious bystander

Although more than 100 years may have passed since natural autoantibodies (NAA) were first identified in human serum (reviewed in [18,19]), how exactly they originate and what specifically is their immunological role still remain a mystery. One explanation is that NAAs are secreted from self-reactive B cells that escape deletion [20] or from immature B cells [21]. Yet, whether they participate in an immune response or maintain immune homeostasis is unknown. It has been suggested that their functions include tumor surveillance, anti-inflammatory activity, first line of defense against infection, antigen presentation to T cells, and clearance of aging cells. NAAs belong to the IgM, IgG, and IgA isotypes, with most of them in adult serum being IgG. Whereas the repertoire of IgG reactivities toward foreign antigens at any age is diverse and dependent upon exposure to pathogens, some studies have noted similar titers of IgG NAAs among infants, young adults and aged individuals. Other studies have shown an increased incidence of NAAs in aged individuals (reviewed in [22]), which thereby makes the relationship between NAAs and autoimmune disease rather ambiguous (unless they protect against these diseases), since the most prevalent and clinically severe autoimmune diseases occur in younger individuals, not in the elderly (reviewed in [18]). One group hypothesized that autoimmune diseases in elderly individuals result from autoantibodies produced by memory B cells that were exposed to self-antigens earlier in life and reactivated later [23].

The role of autoantibodies in developing physiological autoreactivity, pathological autoimmunity and even cancer is yet to be established. Several studies have indicated there may be an inverse correlation between natural antibodies and tumor susceptibility [24]. These results suggest that natural antibodies contribute to resistance against tumors [25]. Some propose that autoantibodies associated with cancer arise from naturally occurring unmutated autoantibody templates through a process of somatic diversification and selection of self-antigens (reviewed in [18]). Since tumor antigens are often modified forms of normal, self-proteins, as isoforms or after undergoing PTMs, anti-tumor antibodies may well be derivatives of NAAs.

Identifying tumor antigens (listed in [26]) is fundamental to finding their cognate antibodies. Tumor antigens are generally divided into several categories (reviewed in [27]). Among these are cancer testis (CT) antigens which have normal expression highly restricted to testis, ovary and placenta, and not other adult somatic tissues, and are abnormally expressed in a wide range of tumors. The list of CT antigens is growing rapidly, with NY-ESO-1 being the most immunogenic known to date, since it induces both a notable humoral and cellular immune response. Serum antibodies to NY-ESO-1 have been detected in melanoma as well as breast, ovarian, lung, esophageal, and bladder cancer (reviewed in [28]). Furthermore, the humoral response could be correlated with clinical events. The titer of anti-NY-ESO-1 autoantibodies decreased upon removal of the tumor or disease regression and increased with progressive disease [29]. These results suggest that NY-ESO-1 antigen expression by the tumor propagates autoantibody production.

Another class of tumor antigens are proteins overexpressed in cancer cells relative to their normal counterparts, such as HER-2/neu in breast cancer. In one study, HER-2/neu antibodies at titers greater than or equal to 1 in 100 were detected in 12 of 107 (11%) breast cancer patients versus none of 200 (0%) normal controls ($P < 0.01$). The presence of antibodies to HER-2/neu also correlated with overexpression of HER-2/neu protein in the patient's primary tumor. This implies that autoantibodies to HER-2/neu develop as a result of exposure to proteins expressed by a patient's own cancer [30].

Several other groups of tumor antigens have been recognized (reviewed in [31]). Defective proteins can be the result of genetic aberrations such as point mutations, truncations, or translocations, as in p53 mutations and lung caner (discussed below). Oncofetal proteins are those that are usually only expressed during fetal development, but then re-expressed during oncogenesis. Carcinoembryonic antigen, which can be highly expressed in colon cancer, is an example. Viral oncogenes associated with chronic infections can lead to cancer, like Epstein-Barr virus leading to B cell lymphoma.

During the carcinogenic process where mutations accumulate and collectively transform normal cells into malignant ones, the mutations may be immunogenic as well as oncogenic (reviewed in [32]). They could create new antigenic epitopes that elicit an autoantibody response, or they could enhance binding of poorly or non-reactive epitopes to antibodies. It has been estimated that mutations to the tumor suppressor p53 are the most frequent genetic event in cancer (reviewed in [33]). Most mutations in p53 increase its half-life from the order of minutes to hours resulting in its pathological accumulation in the nucleus of neoplastic cells. This accumulation has been shown to be the main factor leading to p53 antibody formation. Since normally very small amounts of p53 protein are present in a cell, its abnormal presence (and release from dying cells) is thought to lead to a self-immunization process resulting in p53 antibody formation. Nevertheless, other determinants affect antibody formation since in similar types of cancer with identical mutations and p53 protein accumulation in the nucleus, p53 antibodies are not always generated. About 20–40% of patients with p53 mutations will have p53 antibodies in their serum, which means they could be used for early detection of occult tumors [34]. In one prospective study, two heavy smokers positive for p53 antibodies but negative for any clinically detectable lung cancer were identified. One patient died eight months later from lung cancer, the second was closely followed with p53 antibody assays and chest X-rays. He was diagnosed with lung cancer two years later before any clinical manifestations of the disease were noted. Furthermore, his response to therapy was paralleled by the total disappearance of the p53 antibodies [34,35].

One study assessed whether autoantibodies against an oxidized thymidine molecule, specifically 5-hydroxymethy-2'-deoxyuridine (HMdU), which are significantly higher in chronic inflammatory diseases, could be used to predict breast and colorectal cancer risk. It was found that healthy women at blood donation who were diagnosed 0.5–6 years later with breast or colorectal cancer exhibited statistically significant increased anti-HMdU autoantibody titers over age-matched controls [36]. Another study looked at autoantibodies directed against the M_r 32,000 subunit of replication protein A (RPA32), a protein with a central role in DNA replication, recombination and repair, as possible early markers of ductal breast cancer. Previously it was known that serum antibodies to RPA32 were associated with systemic autoimmune diseases. In this case, anti-RPA32 antibodies were statistically higher among breast cancer patients (87 of 801 patients) than among non-cancer controls (0 of 65). Moreover, these autoantibodies were present in 4 of 39 intraductal *in situ* carcinoma patients, demonstrating their potential use for early detection before the clinical appearance of tumors [37]. All of the aforementioned results show that serum autoantibodies can be detected before clinical manifestations of the disease, suggesting that they are a pathophysiological change manifested very early in the carcinogenic process.

4. Using recombinant expression cloning for identifying tumor antigens as targets for autoantibodies

The two main methodologies for identifying tumor antigens and their cognate antibodies are SEREX and proteomics. SEREX, or serological identification of antigens by recombinant expression cloning, was developed ten years ago as a means of isolating tumor antigens that elicit high-titer IgG responses [38]. The SEREX approach begins by using fresh tumor tissue to construct cDNA λ phage expression libraries. The cDNA libraries are spread onto nitrocellulose membranes and probed with serum from the autologous patient, which has been extensively pre-absorbed to bacterial proteins and diluted (1:100–1:1,000). Clones reactive with high-titre antibodies are isolated and sequenced. Currently, the SEREX database contains nearly 2700 sequences (http://www.licr.org/D_programs/d4ali_SEREX.php).

The initial SEREX study was applied towards four human tumors of different origins, namely malignant melanoma, renal cell carcinoma, astrocytoma and Hodgkin's disease [38]. Their molecular definition of 109 clones containing 24 different inserts conclusively demonstrated that tumors expressed multiple antigens eliciting humoral immune responses in the autologous host. Shortly thereafter, the SEREX technique was extensively used and improved upon to better isolate and define tumor antigens. Applying this method to esophageal squamous cell carcinoma, NY-ESO-1 with its potent humoral and cellular immune reaction, was identified [39]. Numerous studies involving NY-ESO-1 are being conducted, most notably examining the antigens and their/its corresponding humoral response. Another study showed that more than 50% of patients with NY-ESO-1-positive non-small cell lung cancer (NSCLC) develop associated antibodies. Most importantly, they found that NY-ESO-1 antibodies could be detected in patients with small primary tumors and more frequently before distant metastasis occurred [40]. This suggests that these antibodies are formed early on in the process of developing NSCLC and could be used as markers for early detection. On the immunotherapy front, NY-ESO-1 has already been turned into an effective antigen for immunotherapy in a number of cancers, including malignant melanoma, breast cancer and ovarian cancer [41,42].

A few other notable studies using SEREX to identify tumor antigens and autoantibodies are worth mentioning. One study used SEREX to examine glioblastoma multiforme, an aggressive malignant brain tumor. Analyzing serum from 62 patients, they found an autoantibody response against several tumor antigens, specifically GLEA1 in 15 sera (24.2%), GLEA2 in 30 sera (48.4%), and PHF3 in 35 sera (56.5%). They found significantly prolonged survival for patients positive for autoantibodies against GLEA2 ($p = 0.0115$) and PHF3 ($p = 0.0031$), but no correlation for GLEA1 ($p = 0.1611$) [43]. Whether the autoantibodies themselves where the mechanisms underlying the positive prognostic influence or whether they merely represented an effective cellular immune response (or some other immune reaction) was not yet determined.

The Kawakami group used SEREX to look at tumor antigens that induced an immune response in a patient with colorectal cancer. In this case, microsatellite instability caused a frame-shift mutation in the coding region of CDX2, a transcription factor involved in the proliferation and differentiation of intestinal epithelial cells and previously implicated in the development of intestinal tumors. They isolated 64 tumor antigens and detected 49 IgG antibodies when the antigens were probed with the patient's sera compared with that from individuals with various cancers and healthy controls. In particular, they found a tumor-specific IgG antibody response to a mutated form of the CDX2 peptide, which had a unique sequence at its COOH terminus. These CDX2 autoantibodies were no longer detected in the patient's serum seven years after surgical resection, suggesting complete disappearance of the tumors and cure of the patient [44].

There are many advantages of using the SEREX technique (reviewed [45,46]). Using fresh tumor specimens allows for following the expression of *in vivo* genes and avoids artifacts associated with *in vitro* cell lines. Polyclonal antibodies in patient's serum are used as a probe, which allows for the identification of multiple antigens in one course of screening. Since diluted serum is used, only high-titre IgG antibodies are detected which should limit the analysis to those antigens that elicit a strong immune response (and thereby imply cognate T-cell help). cDNA expression cloning facilitates using serological analysis to select clones expressing proteins from all possible cellular compartments, including the cell surface, intracellular proteins and even secreted antigens. The lytic bacteria plaques allow for direct molecular definition of antigens and therefore immediate sequencing and identification, even when starting from the smallest biopsy samples as a source for the mRNAs.

Disadvantages of using SEREX (reviewed in [47]) are related to its innately bias towards detecting anti-gens that are the overexpressed or the result of gene amplification, but not necessarily oncogenic. Often the identified antigens turn out to be patient-specific rather than tumor-specific, and so they do not truly have diagnostic value in clinical practice. Furthermore, since autoantibodies are part of the normal immune system, it can be difficult to isolate those specifically involved in tumorigenesis. Antigens that weakly or do not elicit an antibody response, even if they are highly relevant to carcinogenesis, will go undetected. Similarly, tumor antigens that are the result of PTMs or conformational changes that are either differentially or not expressed in a prokaryotic system will be missed (as will their cognate antibodies). A bacterial expression system is not capable of post-translationally modifying recombinant proteins, and so the conventional SEREX approach will not detect the complete antigen repertoire. As mentioned earlier, tumor antigens often undergo PTMs since these modifications affect protein function and immunogenicity or oncogenicity. A eukaryotic (yeast) expression system was developed for displaying recombinant proteins on the cell surface in a more naturally folded, partially glycosylated manner [48]. They designated their methodology as RAYS, or recombinant antigen expression on yeast surface [49]. Their goal was to search for tumor antigens that could not be detected by conventional prokaryotic expression technologies. Using RAYS, tumor antigens displayed by *Saccharomyces cerevisiae* were probed by autologous and allogenic breast cancer patient serum. Most notably, a variant small breast epithelial mucin (SBEM) protein was isolated, which had previously had gone undetected using SEREX [50]. Although this shows the additive and potentially superior value of RAYS over prokaryotic-based methodologies, SEREX in mammalian cells is still desirable. For example, O-mannosylation of proteins is the dominant PTM in yeast and is essential for cell viability, but it is a less common mammalian protein modification [51].

Even before the RAYS approach, a yeast antibody library expressed in *Saccharomyces cerevisiae* was used [52]. A library of 10^9 human single chain variable fragments (scFv) of antibodies were cloned and expressed on the yeast cell surface. Fluorescence-activated cell sorting (FACS) then allowed for rapid isolation of rare clones with defined binding parameters, and magnetic bead screening facilitated identification of the clones with the highest affinities. The expression, stability, and antigen-binding properties of more than 50 isolated scFv clones were assessed directly on the yeast cell surface without separate subcloning, expression and purification steps. Furthermore, the yeast library could be amplified 10^{10}-fold without measurable loss of clonal diversity, allowing for indefinite expansion. This approach demonstrated that multiplex antibody library screening could be used for high-throughput antibody isolation.

5. Successful proteomics methodologies for identifying tumor antigens and autoantibodies

The main advantage of using proteomics technologies over SEREX to identify tumor antigens and their cognate antibodies is that cancer proteins with PTMs or isoforms of wildtype proteins will be detected. Since proteomics allows for screening tumor proteins in their natural, modified states, the correct conformational epitopes are more likely to be presented for autoantibody recognition and binding. Proteomics technologies allow for examining all of the proteins in a single gel with parallel processing of tumor and normal tissue samples at the same time, unlike SEREX.

Serological proteome analysis, or SERPA, was first applied to renal cell carcinoma (RCC) [1]. The proteomes of non-tumorous kidney and RCC were compared using 2D-PAGE. Five spots were reproducibly reactive with serum from RCC patients and not healthy controls. Two of the spots were isolated and using Edman sequencing and identified as smooth muscle protein 22-α (SM22-α) and an isoform of carbonic anhydrase (CA), CAI. Autoantibodies to the two proteins were detected in serum from 5/11 and 3/11 RCC patients, respectively, whereas serum from 13 healthy individuals did not react. SM22-α was found to be expressed in the mesenchymal cells of the tumor stroma, and not in the malignant RCC cells, possibly due to a tumor-induced stroma reaction. In the course of tumor necrosis, intracellular proteins are released also from mesenchymal cells. Being presented in the context of inflammatory cytokines may have provided the necessary "danger signal" to turn a self-protein into an immunogen resulting in autoantibody formation. The detected isoform of CAI is not usually expressed in non-tumorous kidney, and 2D-PAGE was used to confirm its *de novo* expression in RCC. Interestingly, previous SEREX analysis of RCC identified a different isoform, CAXII, as a tumor associated antigen expressed in about 10% of RCC tumors [38,53]. In that study, CAXII antibodies were detected in the serum of 4/30 RCC patients and 1/30 healthy controls, but not in any of the 30 patients with other cancers (11 with astro-

cytoma and 17 with Hodgkin's disease). As mentioned earlier, one of the major benefits of using SERPA over SEREX is that it uses naturally configured proteins with all of their immunogenic PTMs (reviewed in [1]).

In another study, RCC using a similar approach called SPEAR, or serological and proteomic evaluation of antibody responses [2]. They separated proteins from RCC and normal kidney tissue using 2D-PAGE, and then transferred them to western blots. The blots were probed with sera from the autologous patient and pooled normal serum, instead of multiple individual sera, to eliminate inter-individual variability. Proteins solely reactive with autologous sera were then analyzed using MS. Eleven proteins were identified including CAI, the same tumor antigen found in the SERPA study, and thymidine phosphorylase (TP). In 11/11 of their RCC cases, TP was found to be upregulated with no or minimal expression in normal kidney indicating its potential as a diagnostic marker or therapeutic target.

PROTEOMEX also combined 2D-PAGE with MS to characterize nine metabolic enzymes, which were differentially expressed in RCC compared with normal kidney epithelium [3]. Nine metabolic enzymes were identified for further study, which indicated that a number of biochemical alterations could be associated with RCC, which is probably true of all malignancies. Two isoforms of triosephosphatase isomerase were identified, which were most likely the result of PTMs, and therefore would have gone undetected if proteomics technologies had not been used for the analyses.

Antibody-based Systemic Characterization of Antigens, or Ab SCAN, starts with 1D gel separation of tumor cells and then Western blotting with patient serum to identify proteins of interest. The potential antigens are then identified using MS and genetic profiling [4]. Using Ab SCAN, a novel antigen, mannose-6-phosphate/IGF II receptor, was observed to be the frequent target of humoral immune responses in prostate caner patients. The Ab SCAN approach has several advantages over other methodologies. Running 1D instead of 2D gels, makes the system high-throughput. Less than 0.5 mL of patient serum is needed for the western blot, and all protein bands of interest are simultaneously visualized.

An improved method for transferring proteins separated by 2D-PAGE to a membrane was used in order to screen for and identify antigens recognized by autoantibodies in patients with breast cancer [54]. Their goal was the complete and reproducible recovery of all separated proteins for probing with sera from breast cancer patients and healthy controls. Using MS, they detected three protein isoforms, namely glucose-6-phosphate 1-dehydrogenase, heat shock protein 70, and dihydrolipoyl dehydrogenase, that were preferentially expressed by the breast cancer patients. Furthermore, they concluded that PTMs were responsible for the protein isoforms and therefore the appearance of autoantibodies. They also noticed that the repertoire of IgG autoantibodies are highly conserved between individuals, which supports the idea that most of these are NAAs that can react with a variety of self constituents [55].

During this same time-period, the Hanash group implemented a proteomics approach combining 2D-PAGE with MS for the identification of tumor proteins that elicit a humoral response in a wide variety of cancer patients. They applied their technique to neuroblastoma [56], NSCLC [57,58], breast cancer [59], hepatocellular carcinoma [60], and pancreatic cancer [61].

6. Applying the danger model to tumor antigens and autoantibodies

Scrutinizing all of these studies together, three main conclusions can be drawn. First, although tumor cells have antigens that can be detected using SEREX and proteomics methodologies, an autoantibody response is only elicited in a subset of patients, even among tumors of the same histological subtype. The second recurring theme is that the same antigen and autoantibody can be detected in histologically different cancers. The third point is that several of the same antigens and autoantibodies have been detected in cancers patients as well as those suffering from autoimmune diseases. For example, autoantibodies to heat shock protein 60 (hsp60), a key modulator of protein folding, have been detected in patients with different cancer, individuals with autoimmune disorders, and healthy controls. The hsp60 protein functioning as an antigen with its corresponding autoantibodies have been detected in hepatocellular carcinoma [60], gastric mucosa-associated lymphoid tissue (MALT) lymphoma [62], oral squamous cell carcinoma [63], and osteosarcoma [64]. Several other studies detected hsp60 in association with other types of malignancies, but did not look for an autoantibody response. Not only has hsp60 been associated with a variety of tumors, autoantibodies against it have been reported in the sera of patients with autoimmune disorders such as rheumatoid arthritis [65], diabetes mellitus [65,66], Guillain-Barre syndrome [67], immune thrombocytopenic purpura [68], mixed connective tissue disease, polymyositis/dermatomyositis, pso-

riatic arthritis, inflammatory bowel disease, epidermolysis bullosa acquisita, and bullous pemphigoid [69], and several other disorders.

What combination of factors culminate in humoral immune responses against tumor antigens are yet to be recognized, but they probably are related to factors that vary between individuals. These include major histocompatibility complex (MHC) molecules, blood group antigens, age, gender, health status, and the like (discussed below). Tumor immunogenicity is also variable, since antigenicity unpredictably depends upon protein expression level, processing, PTMs and other factors which are yet to be recognized. Finally, the context of tumor antigen presentation is crucial for eliciting an autoantibody response. The tumor microenvironment can rapidly change depending upon fluctuations in cytokine levels and other immunoregulators causing tumor cell apoptosis and necrosis, or alternatively angiogenesis and metastatic spread.

The danger model [70] offers an explanation for these phenomena by suggesting that the immune system reacts to alarm signals from injured tissues rather than by the recognition of non-self proteins (reviewed in [71]). In this paradigm, healthy cells and even transformed self-cells are being ignored by the immune system because they do not send alarm signals. Therefore, a protein initially associated with a cancer will not be antigenic and elicit an autoantibody response until the surrounding tissue is damaged. Since some autoantibodies are known to be generated early on in the carcinogenic process, initial damage to the tumor microenvironment is probably the cause. On the other hand, some cancers have associated proteins that do not elicit autoantibodies or a detectable immune response, probably because there were never any associated danger signals. This could be one possible explanation why not all patients with a given antigen have a detectable autoantibody response, because the necessary danger signals were not present. Likewise, if normal, healthy tissue gets injured in some way, such that self antigens get presented to the immune system along with danger signals, a pathological autoimmune disorder can result. Although there is no true "danger" to the self, cellular stress or death is inducing a humoral immune response.

In other words, the same heat shock protein (hsp), a normal endogenous protein, can become an antigen in several different ways that involve similar signaling, but result in different pathologies. In cancer, an hsp expressed by a cell that is later transformed into a malignant one becomes antigenic along the way and autoantibodies are formed. Depending on the mutation or aberration, different histological subtypes of cancer can result, explaining how the same hsp can become an antigen associated with different cancers. On the other hand, the same hsp expressed by the same cell that suddenly is in the context of danger signals due to local mechanical damage, toxins, exposure to pathogens or otherwise, can become antigenic with its cognate autoantibodies being formed and cause an autoimmune disease. Thus, any given protein, endogenous or exogenous, can become antigenic and elicit an autoantibody response depending on the context of its presentation.

7. Challenges in developing diagnostic kits

For proteomics research to be reliably developed into early diagnostic kits, several standardization issues need to be resolved (reviewed in [72]). Appropriate specimen handling and proper protein sample preparation are crucial for obtaining accurate and highly reproducible results, since tissue fixation and staining can lead to artifacts. Several techniques for cell disruption and protein extraction exist, and for each cell or tissue type, the optimal method must be evaluated. Proteins and antibodies in serum must be separated from a vast sea of macromolecules and interfering agents, thus making their isolation and purification technically challenging. Prefractionation methods have been developed, but there is always the risk of unintentionally loosing proteins in the process of separating them. Properly identifying proteins from peptides after MS runs would be assisted by multiple sets of data using alternative methods to validate the results.

Although cell lines are often used instead of tumor tissues, caution should always be used in extrapolating results since conditions in culture media may not be representative of the *in vivo* milieu. One study compared proteins from LnCap and PC3, two cell lines, which were derived from patients with metastatic prostate cancer, with individually isolated prostate cancer cells taken from tissue sections. The analysis showed that the *in vitro* and *in vivo* cells shared less than 20% of their proteins [73]. Changes in protein expression occur during long-term and even short-term cell culture due to the artificial conditions associated with "life in plastic". Therefore, extreme caution should be used while attempting to develop early diagnostic kits for cancer purely based on cell lines. Repeated validation with fresh tumor specimens should always be a prerequisite.

Likewise, carcinogenesis in animal models may not always reflect the transformation processes that occur in humans. Although mouse models are extensively used to study malignancies, it may be problematic to extrapolate the experimental results to the human situation. On several occasions, immunotherapies that were deemed successes in animal models were not effective in humans (reviewed in [74]). A novel immunotherapy that was shown to be beneficial in the mouse model for multiple sclerosis, called experimental allergic encephalomyelitis, made it to the clinical trial phase in humans, but the treatments had to be stopped prematurely due to the emergence of a specific population of T cells that correlated with exacerbation of the disease [75]. It could be assumed that the genetic, epigenetic and biochemical mechanisms influencing the immune system and causing cancer in humans differs from those in mice. It is well known that the incidence of cancer rises with advancing age in humans with a dramatic increase in epithelial carcinomas from ages 40 to 80 years old. This is in contrast to most laboratory mouse strains approaching a biologically equivalent age, which develop instead mesenchymal and haematopoietic malignancies (reviewed in [76]). Furthermore, few experiments in tumor immunology are being carried out in old mice, which would be a more appropriate model than younger ones (reviewed in [77]). Consequently, if early diagnostic kits for cancer are developed and tested in mouse models, they would need strict corroboration in humans before wide-scale use.

As mentioned earlier, several factors that vastly differ between individuals could affect their antibody repertoires and would need to be accounted for in order to develop early diagnostic kits that could be used in the general population. Otherwise, binding of antibodies to proteins not associated with the cancer will lead to unacceptable false positive rates. Gender and age differences have been shown to be the cause of differences in autoantibody titres [78]. Autoantibodies to HMdU, the aforementioned oxidized thymidine molecule, were found to be 50% higher in women smokers compared to their male counterparts after adjustment for cigarettes per day. Also, HMdU autoantibodies were significantly elevated in female smokers less than 50 years old, as compared with older female smokers ($p = 0.05$). This could possibly be attributable to cumulative damage from toxins in cigarette smoke and/or from hormonal interactions due to menopausal status and parity. Alternatively, older individuals have an altered B cell repertoire, and therefore may not mount as strong of a humoral immune response. But contradictory evidence shows that with aging there is generally an alteration in the B cell repertoire with an increased serum concentration of autoantibodies (reviewed in [79,80]). This autoantibody increase has been attributed to B cell clonal expansions of two to tenfold, and therefore there is no change in the binding profile of the antibodies and no association with an increased incidence of autoimmune diseases, but there is an increase in B cell neoplasms instead (reviewed in [22]).

Another set of factors affecting the antibody repertoire are inherited traits such as genetic makeup, MHC molecules and blood group antigens. Genetic predisposition to cancer unquestionably exists in some individuals, and being able to use antibodies to detect malignancies early in the course of the disease especially in this population would have a tremendous impact in lowering mortality rates. Interestingly, extremely old people (centenarians in particular) are endowed with a peculiar resistance to cancer (reviewed in [81]), implying that certain genetic factors and possibly the increase in autoantibodies may have a protective effect. Although MHC molecules have been definitively associated with certain autoimmune diseases (reviewed in [82]) and aberrations in their expression have been linked to cancer (reviewed in [83]), how precisely different MHC phenotypes influence the formation of autoantibody repertoires remains to be elucidated. The major and minor blood group antigens clearly affect the antibody repertoire. Antibodies directed against the blood group antigens may result from exposure to carbohydrates that mimic the natural antigens (reviewed in [84]). They also complicate serological proteomics analyses because of cross reactivity between different sources of antigens and of sera. In our laboratory, we used human serum from cancer patients whose blood type was O to probe tumor antigens from cell lines derived from individuals with blood groups A and B. Instead of solely identifying cancer specific antigens and antibodies, we additionally detected reactivity between antibodies and blood group antigens (Hava Segal Masters Thesis and Segal and Admon, in preparation).

Lifestyle choices and habits further influence the antibody repertoire and must be accounted for when devising early detection kits [85]. Occupational exposures, diet, exercise, alcohol consumption, body mass index and vitamins can also evoke, modify or inhibit a humoral immune response. Health status intertwines the autoantibody repertoire with the gamut of pathogen-inducing antibodies. Thus, at any given point in time, each person's serum antibodies are a combination of their NAAs as well as those generated from past exposures to pathogens, environmental toxins, blood transfusions, and medications. The key to successfully devising early detection kits is in separating patient specific versus cancer specific antigens and antibodies, and overcoming the technical challenges associated with developing them into protein and antibody microarrays.

8. The future of humoral proteomics

Proteomics technologies show great promise in facilitating the identification of tumor antigens and their cognate serum antibodies. Specifically, the humoral proteomics approach has shown some early successes in the laboratory, now it is time to translate this potentially powerful tool into early detection kits for cancer. The exquisite inherent sensitivity of serological analysis should be capitalized upon and further developed as a potentially life saving tool. It is only a matter of time before the technical challenges of developing protein and antibody arrays are overcome and early diagnostic kits for cancer and other maladies become a reality.

Acknowledgment

Research in the A. Admon laboratory is funded by the Greta Koppel Small Cell Lung Carcinoma Fund.

References

[1] C.S. Klade, T. Voss, E. Krystek, H. Ahorn, K. Zatloukal, K. Pummer et al., Identification of tumor antigens in renal cell carcinoma by serological proteome analysis, *Proteomics* **1** (2001), 890–898.

[2] R.D. Unwin, P. Harnden, D. Pappin, D. Rahman, P. Whelan, R.A. Craven et al., Serological and proteomic evaluation of antibody responses in the identification of tumor antigens in renal cell carcinoma, *Proteomics* **3** (2003), 45–55.

[3] R. Lichtenfels, R. Kellner, D. Atkins, J. Bukur, A. Ackermann, J. Beck et al., Identification of metabolic enzymes in renal cell carcinoma utilizing PROTEOMEX analyses, *Biochim Biophys Acta* **1646** (2003), 21–31.

[4] Y. Huang, J. Franklin, K. Gifford, B.L. Roberts and C.A. Nicolette, A high-throughput proteo-genomics method to identify antibody targets associated with malignant disease, *Clin Immunol* **111** (2004), 202–209.

[5] Z. Rui, J. Jian-Guo, T. Yuan-Peng, P. Hai and R. Bing-Gen, Use of serological proteomic methods to find biomarkers associated with breast cancer, *Proteomics* **3** (2003), 433–439.

[6] P.H. O'Farrell, High resolution two-dimensional electrophoresis of proteins, *J Biol Chem* **250** (1975), 4007–4021.

[7] R. Aebersold and M. Mann, Mass spectrometry-based proteomics, *Nature* **422** (2003), 198–207.

[8] A. Gorg, W. Postel and S. Gunther, The current state of two-dimensional electrophoresis with immobilized pH gradients, *Electrophoresis* **9** (1988), 531–546.

[9]   F. Chevalier, V. Rofidal, P. Vanova, A. Bergoin and M. Rossignol, Proteomic capacity of recent fluorescent dyes for protein staining, *Phytochemistry* **65** (2004), 1499–506.

[10] W.F. Patton, Detection technologies in proteome analysis, *J Chromatogr B Analyt Technol Biomed Life Sci* **771** (2002), 3–31.

[11] M. Mann, R.C. Hendrickson and A. Pandey, Analysis of proteins and proteomes by mass spectrometry, *Annu Rev Biochem* **70** (2001), 437–473.

[12] A. Pandey and M. Mann, Proteomics to study genes and genomes, *Nature* **405** (2000), 837–846.

[13] J.W. Zolg and H. Langen, How industry is approaching the search for new diagnostic markers and biomarkers, *Mol Cell Proteomics* **3** (2004), 345–354.

[14] V. Espina, A.I. Mehta, M.E. Winters, V. Calvert, J. Wulfkuhle, E.F. Petricoin 3rd, et al., Protein microarrays: molecular profiling technologies for clinical specimens, *Proteomics* **3** (2003), 2091–2100.

[15] H. Zhu and M. Snyder, Protein chip technology, *Curr Opin Chem Biol* **7** (2003), 55–63.

[16] J. Qiu, J. Madoz-Gurpide, D.E. Misek, R. Kuick, D.E. Brenner, G. Michailidis et al., Development of natural protein microarrays for diagnosing cancer based on an antibody response to tumor antigens, *J Proteome Res* **3** (2004), 261–267.

[17] K. Bouwman, J. Qiu, H. Zhou, M. Schotanus, L.A. Mangold, R. Vogt et al. Microarrays of tumor cell derived proteins uncover a distinct pattern of prostate cancer serum immunoreactivity, *Proteomics* **3** (2003), 2200–2207.

[18] S. Lacroix-Desmazes, S.V. Kaveri, L. Mouthon, A. Ayouba, E. Malanchere, A. Coutinho et al., Self-reactive antibodies (natural autoantibodies) in healthy individuals, *Journal of Immunological Methods* **216** (1998), 117–137.

[19] A.B. Poletaev, The immunological homunculus (immunculus) in normal state and pathology, *Biochemistry (Mosc)* **67** (2002), 600–608.

[20] E. Gaudin, Y. Hao, M.M. Rosado, R. Chaby, R. Girard and A.A. Freitas, Positive selection of B cells expressing low densities of self-reactive BCRs, *J Exp Med* **199** (2004), 843–853.

[21] H. Wardemann, S. Yurasov, A. Schaefer, J.W. Young, E. Meffre and M.C. Nussenzweig, Predominant autoantibody production by early human B cell precursors, *Science* **301** (2003), 1374–1277.

[22] M.E. Weksler and P. Szabo, The effect of age on the B-cell repertoire, *J Clin Immunol* **20** (2000), 240–249.

[23] S. Stacy, K.A. Krolick, A.J. Infante and E. Kraig, Immunological memory and late onset autoimmunity, *Mech Ageing Dev* **123** (2002), 975–985.

[24] R.D. Bennet and D.A. Chow, Inverse correlation between natural antitumor antibodies and tumor susceptibility in individual xid-bearing mice, *Nat Immun Cell Growth Regul* **10** (1991), 45–55.

[25] D.A. Chow and R.D. Bennet, Low natural antibody and low in vivo tumor resistance, in xid-bearing B-cell deficient mice, *J Immunol* **142** (1989), 3702–3706.

[26] L. Novellino, C. Castelli and G. Parmiani, A listing of human tumor antigens recognized by T cells: March 2004 update, *Cancer Immunol Immunother* **7** (2004), 187–207.

[27] L. Radvanyi, Discovery and immunologic validation of new antigens for therapeutic cancer vaccines, *Int Arch Allergy Immunol* **133** (2004), 179–197.

[28] M.J. Scanlan, A.O. Gure, A.A. Jungbluth, L.J. Old and Y.T. Chen, Cancer/testis antigens: an expanding family of targets for cancer immunotherapy, *Immunol Rev* **188** (2002), 22–32.

[29] E. Jager, E. Stockert, Z. Zidianakis, Y.T. Chen, J. Karbach, D. Jager et al., Humoral immune responses of cancer patients against Cancer-Testis antigen NY-ESO-1: correlation with clinical events, *Int J Cancer* **84** (1999), 506–510.

[30] M.L. Disis, S.M. Pupa, J.R. Gralow, R. Dittadi, S. Menard and M.A. Cheever, High-titer HER-2/neu protein-specific antibody can be detected in patients with early-stage breast cancer, *J Clin Oncol* **15** (1997), 3363–3367.

[31] J.A. Berzofsky, M. Terabe, S. Oh, I.M. Belyakov, J.D. Ahlers, J.E. Janik et al., Progress on new vaccine strategies for the immunotherapy and prevention of cancer, *J Clin Invest* **113** (2004), 1515–1525.

[32] M.J. Turk, J.D. Wolchok, J.A. Guevara-Patino, S.M. Goldberg and A.N. Houghton, Multiple pathways to tumor immunity and concomitant autoimmunity, *Immunol Rev* **188** (2002), 122–135.

[33] T. Soussi, p53 Antibodies in the sera of patients with various types of cancer: a review, *Cancer Res* **60** (2000), 1777–1788.

[34] R. Lubin, G. Zalcman, L. Bouchet, J. Tredanel, Y. Legros, D. Cazals et al., Serum p53 antibodies as early markers of lung cancer, *Nat Med* **1** (1995), 701–702.

[35] G. Zalcman, B. Schlichtholz, J. Tredaniel, T. Urban, R. Lubin, I. Dubois et al., Monitoring of p53 autoantibodies in lung cancer during therapy: relationship to response to treatment, *Clin Cancer Res* **4** (1998), 1359–1366.

[36] K. Frenkel, J. Karkoszka, T. Glassman, N. Dubin, P. Toniolo, E. Taioli et al., Serum autoantibodies recognizing 5-hydroxymethyl-2'-deoxyuridine, an oxidized DNA base, as biomarkers of cancer risk in women, *Cancer Epidemiol Biomarkers Prev* **7** (1998), 49–57.

[37] J.E. Tomkiel, H. Alansari, N. Tang, J.B. Virgin, X. Yang, P. VandeVord et al., Autoimmunity to the M(r) 32,000 subunit of replication protein A in breast cancer, *Clin Cancer Res* **8** (2002), 752–758.

[38] U. Sahin, O. Tureci, H. Schmitt, B. Cochlovius, T. Johannes, R. Schmits et al., Human neoplasms elicit multiple specific immune responses in the autologous host, *Proc Natl Acad Sci USA* **92** (1995), 11810–11813.

[39] Y.T. Chen, M.J. Scanlan, U. Sahin, O. Tureci, A.O. Gure, S. Tsang et al., A testicular antigen aberrantly expressed in human cancers detected by autologous antibody screening, *Proc Natl Acad Sci USA* **94** (1997), 1914–1918.

[40] O. Tureci, U. Mack, U. Luxemburger, H. Heinen, F. Krummenauer, M. Sester et al., Humoral immune responses of lung cancer patients against tumor antigen NY-ESO-1, *Cancer Lett* (2005), 64–71.

[41] E. Jager, S. Gnjatic, Y. Nagata, E. Stockert, D. Jager, J. Karbach et al., Induction of primary NY-ESO-1 immunity: CD8+ T lymphocyte and antibody responses in peptide-vaccinated patients with NY-ESO-1+ cancers. *Proc Natl Acad Sci USA* **97** (2000), 12198–203.

[42] R.F. Wang, S.L. Johnston, G. Zeng, S.L. Topalian, D.J. Schwartzentruber and S.A. Rosenberg, A breast and melanoma-shared tumor antigen: T cell responses to antigenic peptides translated from different open reading frames, *J Immunol* **161** (1998), 3598–3606.

[43] C.P. Pallasch, A.K. Struss, A. Munnia, J. Konig, W.I. Steudel, U. Fischer et al., Autoantibodies against GLEA2 and PHF3 in glioblastoma: Tumor-associated autoantibodies correlated with prolonged survival. *International Journal of Cancer* (2005), 456–459.

[44] T. Ishikawa, T. Fujita, Y. Suzuki, S. Okabe, Y. Yuasa, T. Iwai et al., Tumor-specific immunological recognition of frameshift-

mutated peptides in colon cancer with microsatellite instability, *Cancer Res* **63** (2003), 5564–5572.

[45] G. Li, A. Miles, A. Line and R.C. Rees, Identification of tumour antigens by serological analysis of cDNA expression cloning, *Cancer Immunol Immunother* **53** (2004), 139–143.

[46] O. Tureci, U. Sahin and M. Pfreundschuh, Serological analysis of human tumor antigens: molecular definition and implications, *Mol Med Today* **3** (1997), 342–349.

[47] F. Fernandez Madrid, N. Tang, H. Alansari, R.L. Karvonen and J.E. Tomkiel, Improved approach to identify cancer-associated autoantigens, *Autoimmun Rev* **4** (2005), 230–235.

[48] E.T. Boder and K.D. Wittrup, Yeast surface display for screening combinatorial polypeptide libraries, *Nat Biotechnol* **15** (1997), 553–557.

[49] A. Mischo, A. Wadle, K. Watzig, D. Jager, E. Stockert, D. Santiago et al., Recombinant antigen expression on yeast surface (RAYS) for the detection of serological immune responses in cancer patients, *Cancer Immun* **3** (2003), 5.

[50] A. Wadle, A. Mischo, J. Imig, B. Wullner, D. Hensel, K. Watzig et al., Serological identification of breast cancer-related antigens from a Saccharomyces cerevisiae surface display library, *Int J Cancer* **117** (2005), 104–113.

[51] T. Willer, M.C. Valero, W. Tanner, J. Cruces and S. Strahl, O-mannosyl glycans: from yeast to novel associations with human disease, *Curr Opin Struct Biol* **13** (2003), 621–630.

[52] M.J. Feldhaus, R.W. Siegel, L.K. Opresko, J.R. Coleman, J.M. Feldhaus, Y.A. Yeung et al., Flow-cytometric isolation of human antibodies from a nonimmune Saccharomyces cerevisiae surface display library, *Nat Biotechnol* **21** (2003), 163–170.

[53] O. Tureci, U. Sahin, E. Vollmar, S. Siemer, E. Gottert, G. Seitz et al., Human carbonic anhydrase XII: cDNA cloning, expression, and chromosomal localization of a carbonic anhydrase gene that is overexpressed in some renal cell cancers, *Proc Natl Acad Sci USA* **95** (1998), 7608–7613.

[54] L. Canelle, J. Bousquet, C. Pionneau, L. Deneux, N. Imam-Sghiouar, M. Caron et al., An efficient proteomics-based approach for the screening of autoantibodies, *Journal of Immunological Methods* **299** (2005), 77–89.

[55] S. Avrameas and T. Ternynck, Natural autoantibodies: the other side of the immune system, *Res Immunol* **146** (1995), 235–248.

[56] L. Prasannan, D.E. Misek, R. Hinderer, J. Michon, J.D. Geiger and S.M. Hanash, Identification of beta-tubulin isoforms as tumor antigens in neuroblastoma, *Clin Cancer Res* **6** (2000), 3949–3956.

[57] F. Brichory, D. Beer, F. Le Naour, T. Giordano and S. Hanash, Proteomics-based identification of protein gene product 9.5 as a tumor antigen that induces a humoral immune response in lung cancer, *Cancer Res* **61** (2001), 7908–7912.

[58] F.M. Brichory, D.E. Misek, A.M. Yim, M.C. Krause, T.J. Giordano, D.G. Beer et al., An immune response manifested by the common occurrence of annexins I and II autoantibodies and high circulating levels of IL-6 in lung cancer, *Proc Natl Acad Sci USA* **98** (2001), 9824–9829.

[59] F. Le Naour, D.E. Misek, M.C. Krause, L. Deneux, T.J. Giordano, S. Scholl et al., Proteomics-based identification of RS/DJ-1 as a novel circulating tumor antigen in breast cancer, *Clin Cancer Res* **7** (2001), 3328–3335.

[60] F. Le Naour, F. Brichory, D.E. Misek, C. Brechot, S.M. Hanash and L. Beretta, A distinct repertoire of autoantibodies in hepatocellular carcinoma identified by proteomic analysis, *Mol Cell Proteomics* **1** (2002), 197–203.

[61] S.H. Hong, D.E. Misek, H. Wang, E. Puravs, T.J. Giordano, J.K. Greenson et al., An autoantibody-mediated immune response to calreticulin isoforms in pancreatic cancer, *Cancer Res* **64** (2004), 5504–5510.

[62] E. Ishii, K. Yokota, T. Sugiyama, Y. Fujinaga, K. Ayada, I. Hokari et al., Immunoglobulin G1 antibody response to Helicobacter pylori heat shock protein 60 is closely associated with low-grade gastric mucosa-associated lymphoid tissue lymphoma, *Clin Diagn Lab Immunol* **8** (2001), 1056–1059.

[63] M. Castelli, F. Cianfriglia, A. Manieri, L. Palma, R.W. Pezzuto, G. Falasca et al., Anti-p53 and anti-heat shock proteins antibodies in patients with malignant or pre-malignant lesions of the oral cavity. *Anticancer Res* **21** (2001), 753–758.

[64] K. Trieb, R. Gerth, R. Windhager, J.G. Grohs, G. Holzer, P. Berger et al., Serum antibodies against the heat shock protein 60 are elevated in patients with osteosarcoma, *Immunobiology* **201** (2000), 368–376.

[65] Y. Ozawa, A. Kasuga, H. Nomaguchi, T. Maruyama, T. Kasatani, A. Shimada et al., Detection of autoantibodies to the pancreatic islet heat shock protein 60 in insulin-dependent diabetes mellitus, *J Autoimmun* **9** (1996), 517–524.

[66] L. Koranyi, E. Hegedus, E. Peterfal and I. Kurucz, [The role of hsp60 and hsp70 kDa heat shock protein families in different types of diabetes mellitus], *Orv Hetil* **145** (2004), 467–472.

[67] K. Yonekura, S. Yokota, S. Tanaka, H. Kubota, N. Fujii, H. Matsumoto et al., Prevalence of anti-heat shock protein antibodies in cerebrospinal fluids of patients with Guillain-Barre syndrome, *J Neuroimmunol* **156** (2004), 204–209.

[68] C. Xiao, S. Chen, M. Yuan, F. Ding, D. Yang, R. Wang et al., Expression of the 60 kDa and 71 kDa heat shock proteins and presence of antibodies against the 71 kDa heat shock protein in pediatric patients with immune thrombocytopenic purpura, *BMC Blood Disord* **4** (2004), 1.

[69] W.N. Jarjour, B.D. Jeffries, J.St. Davis, W.J. Welch, T. Mimura and J.B. Winfield, Autoantibodies to human stress proteins. A survey of various rheumatic and other inflammatory diseases, *Arthritis Rheum* **34** (1991), 1133–1138

[70] P. Matzinger, Tolerance, danger, and the extended family, *Annu Rev Immunol* **12** (1994), 991–1045.

[71] P. Matzinger, The danger model: a renewed sense of self, *Science* **296** (2002), 301–305.

[72] S.H. Shoshan and A. Admon, Proteomics in clinical laboratory diagnosis, *Adv Clin Chem* **39** (2005), 159–184.

[73] D.K. Ornstein, J.W. Gillespie, C.P. Paweletz, P.H. Duray, J. Herring, C.D. Vocke et al., Proteomic analysis of laser capture microdissected human prostate cancer and in vitro prostate cell lines, *Electrophoresis* **21** (2000), 2235–2242.

[74] S.A. Rosenberg, Shedding light on immunotherapy for cancer, *N Engl J Med* **350** (2004), 1461–1463.

[75] B. Bielekova, B. Goodwin, N. Richert, I. Cortese, T. Kondo, G. Afshar et al., Encephalitogenic potential of the myelin basic protein peptide (amino acids 83–99) in multiple sclerosis: results of a phase II clinical trial with an altered peptide ligand, *Nat Med* **6** (2000), 1167–1175.

[76] R.A. DePinho, The age of cancer, *Nature* **408** (2000), 248–254.

[77] O.J. Finn, Tumor immunology at the service of cancer immunotherapy, *Curr Opin Immunol* **16** (2004), 127–129.

[78] L.A. Mooney, F.P. Perera, A.M. Van Bennekum, W.S. Blaner, J. Karkoszka, L. Covey et al., Gender differences in autoantibodies to oxidative DNA base damage in cigarette smokers, *Cancer Epidemiol Biomarkers Prev* **10** (2001), 641–648.

[79] G. Colonna-Romano, M. Bulati, A. Aquino, G. Scialabba, G. Candore, D. Lio et al., B cells in the aged: CD27, CD5, and CD40 expression, *Mech Ageing Dev* **124** (2003), 389–393.

[80] F.T. Hakim, F.A. Flomerfelt, M. Boyiadzis and R.E. Gress, Aging, immunity and cancer, *Curr Opin Immunol* **16** (2004), 151–156.

[81] M. Bonafe, S. Valensin, W. Gianni, V. Marigliano and C. Franceschi, The unexpected contribution of immunosenescence to the leveling off of cancer incidence and mortality in the oldest old, *Crit Rev Oncol Hematol* **39** (2001), 227–233.

[82] S.H. Shoshan and A. Admon, MHC-bound antigens and proteomics for novel target discovery, *Pharmacogenomics* **5** (2004), 845–859.

[83] A. Garcia-Lora, I. Algarra, A. Collado and F. Garrido, Tumour immunology, vaccination and escape strategies, *Eur J Immunogenet* **30** (2003), 177–183.

[84] A. Pruss, A. Salama, N. Ahrens, A. Hansen, H. Kiesewetter, J. Koscielny et al., Immune hemolysis-serological and clinical aspects, *Clin Exp Med* **3** (2003), 55–64.

[85] P. Wallstrom, K. Frenkel, E. Wirfalt, B. Gullberg, J. Karkoszka, J. Seidegard et al., Antibodies against 5-hydroxymethyl-2'-deoxyuridine are associated with lifestyle factors and GSTM1 genotype: a report from the Malmo Diet and Cancer cohort, *Cancer Epidemiol Biomarkers Prev* **12** (2003), 444–451.

Cancer Biomarkers 3 (2007) 153–161
IOS Press

Cyclooxygenase-2 as target for chemopreventive interventions: New approaches

Hadas Dvory-Sobol and Nadir Arber*
Integrated Cancer Prevention Center, Tel Aviv Medical Center and Sackler School of Medicine, Tel Aviv University, Israel

Abstract. Preventive medicine has become a corner stone in our concept of health in the third millennium. Colorectal cancer (CRC) fits the criteria of a disease suitable for prevention interventions. This is a prevalent disease that is associated with considerable mortality and morbidity rates. More than 1,000,000 new cases and 500,000 deaths are expected, worldwide, in 2005. CRC has a natural history of transition from precursor to malignant lesion that spans, on average, 15–20 years, providing a window of opportunity for effective interventions and prevention. A pre-malignant precursor lesion (i.e., adenoma) usually precedes cancer, and helps to identify a subset of the population that is at increased risk of harboring and developing cancer. Science and technology have evolved to a point where we are able to use our knowledge of cancer biology to identify individuals at risk. Since compliance with current screening methods is a major barrier to the achievement of optimal results, a large part of the average risk population has not been screened by any method. Hence, chemoprevention, a new science that has emerged during the last decade, presents an alternative approach to reducing mortality from CRC.

Keywords: Colorectal cancer, chemoprevention, cyclooxygenase, curcumin

1. Introduction

The famed surgeon Dr. Billroth once said that cancer could be cured with a knife [1]. Dr. Billroth was later proven wrong. Despite advances in surgery, radiation therapy and chemotherapy, cancer surpassed heart disease and became the leading cause of death in the western world [1]. Therefore, at the dawn of this century, cancer prevention is the new frontier for cancer therapy.

Colorectal cancer (CRC) is a leading cause of cancer-related death in the western world. Incidence and mortality from CRC are similar in both men and women [2]. In women, CRC ranks third after lung and breast cancer, while in men, it ranks third after lung and prostate cancer. The incidence of CRC increases sharply after the age of 50 and the estimated lifetime risk is 5% to 6%. Approximately 75% of new cases occur in individuals at average risk [2,3]. Because of the high incidence of the cancer, with more than one million new cases expected worldwide in 2005, and the considerable mortality and morbidity associated, with about 500,000 deaths expected worldwide in the same year [4,5], the prevention of CRC has become an important public health goal. The past two decades have seen the emergence of chemopreventive agents that have one of three effects: inhibiting, delaying, or reversing carcinogenesis. Recent data from the World Health Organization indicate that CRC has reached the highest incidence of all malignancies in Europe [5,6].

Strategies to improve survival and reduce mortality from this disease focus on prevention, early detection and improvement of current therapy.

CRC is preventable in up to 80–90% of the cases. Life style modifications are particularly important as

<hr>

*Corresponding author: Prof. Nadir Arber, Head – Integrated Cancer Prevention Center, Tel-Aviv Medical Center, 6 Weizmann St., Tel-Aviv 64239, Israel. Tel.: +1 972 3 6974968; Fax: +1 972 3 6950339; E-mail: nadir@tasmc.health.gov.il; narber@post.tau.ac.il.

they can prevent other diseases as well. The most significant life style habits are a regular exercise regime, a healthy diet and abstinence from smoking and drinking.

The International Agency for Research on Cancer (IARC; part of WHO) uses the term chemoprevention to refer to interventions with pharmaceuticals, vitamins, minerals or other chemicals (natural or synthetic) at any of the multiple stages of carcinogenesis to reduce cancer incidence [7].

Chemoprevention science has emerged during the last decade, and presents an alternative approach to reducing mortality from CRC [8–10]. In CRC, chemoprevention involves the long-term use of a variety of oral agents that can delay, prevent or even reverse the development of adenomas in the large bowel and interfere with the multi-step progression from adenoma to carcinoma.

Chemoprevention is of particular importance to genetically predisposed patients and to those patients who are especially susceptible to the environmental causes of CRC.

The ideal chemopreventive agent should fulfill the following criteria:

1. The drug must be effective;
2. It should have a convenient dosing schedule of not more than once a day;
3. It should be easily administered;
4. It should have no side effects, or a very low side effect profile in high risk populations; and
5. It should have a low cost

Recent observations suggest a number of potential targets for chemoprevention. Although many compounds and agents have potential benefits, their chemopreventive efficacy in clinical trials has been modest (20%). Non-steroidal anti-inflammatory drugs (NSAIDs), on the other hand, can prevent cancer in approximately 50% of the cases.

2. NSAIDs and CRC

The association between NSAIDs and CRC is intriguing and comprehensive. The discovery of the potential chemopreventive activity of NSAIDs in sporadic human CRC, almost 20 years ago, represents an important example of chemoprevention [11,12]. In fact, observations suggesting that NSAIDs reduce the incidence and mortality from CRC are supported by the results of more than 100 well-conducted, randomized, double blind, placebo-controlled animal studies,

in which the administration of various NSAIDs consistently resulted in fewer tumors per animal and fewer animals with tumors, clearly demonstrating the preventive effect of NSAIDs on carcinogen-induced colorectal tumorgenesis in rodents [13,14]. Intervention data in familial adenomatous polyposis (FAP) have established that NSAIDs exert their effect on the process of human colonic adenoma formation [15]. Supportive evidence for the role NSAIDs in the prevention of CRC was also derived from 33 of 35 epidemiological studies (both case-control and cohort), that found a reduced risk in men and women, treated with NSAIDs, for cancers of the colon and the rectum. The protective effect is dose dependant, and more importantly, is directly related to the duration of exposure [12,15–17].

It is estimated that at least 20 to 30 billion aspirin tablets are purchased annually in the United States alone, and that 1% to 2% of the world population consumes at least one aspirin tablet daily [18]. At present there are at least 15 NSAIDs on the market, being prescribed at a rate of 70 million NSAID prescriptions per year for individuals suffering from chronic inflammation and pain; for example 10 to 15 million individuals afflicted with rheumatoid arthritis (RA) and osteoarthritis in the United States [19].

Unfortunately, while taking aspirin, sulindac and other older NSAIDS reduce the incidence and mortality from CRC, their chronic use is not problem-free, and can cause serious life-threatening gastro-intestinal complications. In 1997, 107,000 hospitalizations and 16,500 deaths, in the United States alone, were due to NSAIDs consumption [19]. Therefore, although chemoprevention of CRC is already possible, drugs that have more acceptable side-effect profiles than the currently available NSAIDs are required.

3. Mechanism of action: Traditional and new generation of NSAIDs

Traditional NSAIDs inhibit both cyclooxygenase 1 (COX-1), by irreversible acetylation, and cyclooxygenase 2 (COX-2), by competitive inhibition [20]. However, while COX-2 is usually elevated in 40% of colorectal adenomas and in up to 85% of CRC (but not in normal gastrointestinal mucosa) [21,22], COX-1 serves as a housekeeping protein which is required for physiological processes such as the maintenance of the gastrointestinal mucosa and platelet aggregation.

Oncogenes, growth factors, cytokines, chemotherapeutics, and tumor promoters are among some of the stimuli that induce COX-2 expression. COX-2 induction has been associated with various pre-malignant and malignant lesions of epithelial origin in organs such as colon, lung, breast, prostate, bladder, stomach, and esophagus (reviewed in Dannenberg et al. [23]). Although the underlying mechanisms of this elevated COX-2 expression in cancer is not known, key *cis*-acting elements within the promoter of the COX-2 gene have been shown to play an important role in the regulation of COX-2. The promoter region of COX-2 consists of many transcription factor binding sites, such as nuclear factor κB (NFκB), nuclear factor of interleukin-6 (NF-IL-6), cyclic adenosine monophosphate (cAMP) response element (CRE) and hypoxia-inducible factor-1 (HIF-1); most of which are known to be involved in the up-regulation of COX-2 by inflammatory stimuli or tumor promoters (reviewed in Dempke et al. [24]). It has been hypothesized that the up-regulation of COX-2 prolongs the survival of abnormal cells and thereby favors the accumulation of sequential genetic changes, which increases the risk of tumorgenesis [25].

Concerning CRC, Eberhart et al. [26] were the first to identify significant elevations of COX-2 expression in 85% and 50% of human colorectal carcinomas and adenomas respectively. In normal intestinal tissue, immuno-localization studies have shown the expression of both COX-1 and COX-2 in mucosal epithelial cells, mononuclear cells, vascular endothelial cells and smooth muscle [27]. However, in both human and animal models of colorectal cancers, COX-2 expression is dramatically increased in malignancies when compared with adjacent normal mucosa [28]. COX-1 expression appears to remain unaltered or even reduced [29].

Consequently, by inhibiting COX-1, non-selective NSAIDs abrogate a series of key prostaglandin defense mechanisms which result in toxicity that is expressed in the gastrointestinal and renal mucosa. The side effects associated with the dual COX-inhibitory effect of traditional NSAIDs meant that physicians were reluctant to adopt their widespread use for the prevention of CRC. To diminish the side effects of traditional NSAIDs, a new class of NSAIDs was developed to selectively inhibit COX-2 and not COX-1. Aspirin is an irreversible inhibitor of the COX active site. It covalently modifies the COX protein by acetylating a single serine residue in the substrate-binding channel, blocking the approach of arachidonic acid. Indomethacin, piroxicam, ibuprofen, and sulindac are competitive inhibitors that non-covalently bind to the protein in the substrate channel. The structural differences between COX-1 and COX-2 have been exploited by pharmaceutical companies to develop selective COX-2 inhibitors [30–32]. The active site of COX-2 is larger than that of COX-1 with an additional side-pocket (31) that can accommodate larger structures. The replacement of isoleucine by valine in the binding site of COX-1, for example, removes constriction in the mouth of this secondary pocket, which results in access by more bulky molecules [31]. This class of selective COX-2 inhibitors which has an improved safety profile [33] offers the benefits of cancer protection without the gastrointestinal toxicity and platelet dysfunction that was reported for the "old" NSAIDs; it is particularly important in chemoprevention studies, which may be long term in nature and involve healthy subjects and minimal toxicity. The inhibition of the growth of pre-cancerous and cancerous cells without affecting normal cells is also the ultimate aim of cancer treatment.

Three International multi-center, prospective, randomized, placebo-controlled trials studying a secondary prevention of CRC were launched in the years 1999 and 2000, in order to evaluate the efficacy of celecoxib and rofecoxib in the secondary prevention of colorectal polyps [36,37]. Each study recruited between 1,500 to 2,500 patients from over 100 sites. The primary endpoint was the number of patients with adenomatous polyps. The Adenomatous Polyp Prevention on Vioxx (APPROVe) trial recruited 2586 patients with a history of colorectal adenomas. They received 25 mg of rofecoxib daily ($n = 1257$) or placebo ($n = 1299$) for three year [37]. A 25% reduction in adenomas recurrence was found in the treatment group. The Adenoma Prevention with Celecoxib (APC) trial included 2,026 patients, with randomization to either placebo or celecoxib (200 or 400 mg twice daily) in a large CRC prevention clinical trial. The patients had an adenomatous polyp removed before enrollment and were followed-up for a mean of 33 months while taking the study drug. Follow at 3 years found a significant reduction in polyp recurrence ($p < 0.0001$) [38]. The PreSAP (Prevention of Sporadic Adenomatous Polyps) trial was conducted in parallel to the APC trial for the same indication. One thousand sixty one patients with a history of colorectal adenomas were randomized 3:2 to receive either 400 mg celecoxib daily or placebo. Polyp recurrence rate was 33% in the celecoxib group vs 49.3% in the placebo group ($p < 0.0001$) [39,40]. All three trials found that selective COX-2 inhibitors may reduce polyp recurrence in the sporadic setting, however, in the APPROVe and the APC study this was associated with an increase risk of cardiovascular events (mainly myocardial infarction, stroke, and heart failure) [37].

On September 25 2004, Merck dramatically announced the early termination of their study. Vioxx was withdrawn from the market due to increased cardiovascular toxicity in patients receiving the drug for more than 18 months. A total of 46 patients in the rofecoxib group had a confirmed thrombotic event compared with 26 patients in the placebo group (RR: 1.92). On December 17, 2004, the National Cancer Institute suspended the APC trial. The study was stopped because analysis by an independent adjudication cardiovascular committee, a subcommittee of its Data Safety and Monitoring Board, showed a significant dose-response excess of major cardiovascular events of 2.5 and 3.5 for the celecoxib 200 and 400 mg bid groups compared to the placebo group [36]. At the same time, in the PreSAP trial the RR of celecoxib 400 mg qd group compared to the placebo group was non-significant at 1.3 [40].

While short term use of these agents seems to be safe chronic use as necessary for achieving the goals of chemoprevention carries a cardiovascular hazard and determining specific sub-populations who may benefit from these drugs vs populations who are at increased risk for these side effects remains an important and open question. These studies confirm an association between the COX-2 enzyme and development of colonic adenomas. They provide a proof of concept for an important step toward developing effective colorectal cancer prevention. It also shows that selective COX-2 inhibitors must be use cautiously, particularly for patients with a history of cardiovascular disease.

The message of these trials is that selective COX-2 inhibitors are highly effective agents for prevention of pre-cancerous lesions of the colon. At the same time, although relatively safe in terms of gastrointestinal (GI) toxicity, their use in the setting of CRC prevention carries a risk of serious cardiovascular complications. As a result, they cannot be routinely recommended for colorectal cancer prevention in the entire population.

4. Other mechanism involve in the protective effects of NSAIDs

The molecular mechanism responsible for the chemopreventive action of NSAIDs is not completely clear. Candidate targets are key proteins in the cell cycle and the apoptotic process. Regulation of angiogenesis is another mechanisms for the decreased colon carcinogenesis associated with the inhibition of COX-2 [41,42]. However, because cells that do not express COX-2 also undergo apoptosis in response to NSAIDs,

it is also possible that these drugs act by COX-2 independent mechanisms such as the inhibition of the activity of nuclear factor kB, interference with the binding of the peroxisome proliferators delta (PPAR-δ) to DNA, activation of PPAR-γ, activation of protein kinase G and down-regulation of the anti-apoptotic protein Bcl-XL [43–46]. The presence of multiple molecular targets offers the potential for combination therapies, which may be more effective than any agent alone. This is of particular importance since one of the lessons learned from cancer research in recent decades is that combinatorial strategies for cancer therapy can provide dramatic improvement in safety and efficacy over mono-therapeutic regiments, especially if the combined drugs differ in their mode of action.

5. Curcumin, a multi-functional chemopreventive agent

Curcumin (diferuloylmethane), a natural plant product, possesses chemopreventive activity that targets multiple signaling pathways in the prevention of CRC development. The therapeutic benefits of curcumin have been reported as an analgesic, anticoagulant, antibacterial, antiviral, anti-parasitic, antioxidant, antiarthritic, anti-hypercholesterolemic, antihypertensive, carminative, and depurature. There are at least six phase I human trials showing the safety and of curcumin in humans [47]. Since curcumin has been classified as a chemopreventive agent, a particular interest arises in its ability to interfere with colon carcinogenesis in chemical and genetic rodent models [48–50]. Dietary curcumin has been shown to prevent CRC in mice [51]. Furthermore, curcumin has also been associated with the regression of established malignancy in humans [52]. It specifically inhibits cyclooxygenase-2 (COX-2) expression, which plays an important role in CRC carcinogenesis [53–55]. It appears that curcumin can inhibit cell growth by inhibiting cellular protein kinases, such as protein kinase C (PKC), c-Jun terminal kinase (JNK), and the epidermal growth factor (EGF) receptor kinase [56,57]. Curcumin also has a profound ability to block the NF-κB cell survival pathway [58]. A study of the clinical application of curcumin as a chemopreventive agent was intensively carried out at the National Cancer Institute [54].

Recently, we have shown that curcumin potentiates the growth inhibitory effect of celecoxib by shifting the dose-response curve to the left. The synergistic growth inhibition effect was mediated through a mechanism that probably involves inhibition of COX-2 pathway and may involve other non-COX-2 pathways [59]. This synergistic effect is clinically important since it can be achieved in the serum of patients receiving standard anti-inflammatory or anti-neoplastic dosages of celecoxib. Similarly, we have shown a synergistic growth inhibition of pancreatic cells *in vitro* [60]. A phase III trial of conventional therapy ± curcumin and celecoxib in the setting of un-resectable pancreatic cancer and metastatic CRC had received an IRB approval and will soon start to recruit patients.

6. COX-2 and NF-κB activation

As indicated earlier, NF-κB is a nuclear target of the intracellular pathways that lead to COX-2 expression and is a positive regulator of COX-2 in many cell types [65] Tumor promoters such as arsenic have been reported to induce COX-2 transcription mediated through activation of IκB kinase and NF-κB activities [66]. Two putative NF-κB binding sites are found in the 5/ promoter region of COX-2 and activation of NF-κB results in translocation of NF-κB to the nucleus, where it can bind to one of two *cis*-acting elements in the promoter region of COX-2 [66]. Besides NF-κB, AP-1 is also implicated in COX-2 transcriptional activation [67] and induction of COX-2 is at least partially mediated by MAP kinases. This idea is further supported by findings showing that the induction of COX-2 and/or resulting prostaglandin production was abolished by inhibition of MAP kinases [68,69].

7. Chemoprevention and other dietary factors

7.1. Cox-2 and n-3 fatty acids

It has been shown that n-3 polyunsaturated fatty acids, DHA and EPA, effectively reduced the tumor number and tumor growth particularly in the small intestine, but also in the colon in Min mice. In addition a reduced number of AFC in the min mice was recorded in the colon [65]. DHA reduced the intestinal tumor number in the ApcΔ716 [66]. The mechanisms could be that DHA inhibits COX-2 and EPA competes with arachidonic acid giving rise to accumulation of arachidonic acid, which may stimulate apoptosis [67] and less active leukotriens and prostaglandins [68,69].

7.2. Resveratrol and COX-2

The inhibitory effect of resveratrol on COX-2 has been proposed as one of the major mechanisms for its anti-cancer effects [70]. In the NMBA-induced rat esophageal tumorgenesis model, resveratrol treatment resulted in a significantly decreased number and mean volume of tumors compared to NMBA-treated only groups [71]. Treatment with resveratrol suppressed the NMBA-induced expression of COX-2 and production of prostaglandin E2 (PGE$_2$) [74]. Resveratrol may also affect other pathways besides NF-κB that would lead to a down-regulation of COX-2. Resveratrol inhibited both COX-2 enzyme activity and phorbol ester-induced activation (PMA) of COX-2, which appeared to occur through a suppression of PMA-dependent activation of protein kinase C (PKC) and AP-1 mediated gene expression [72]. These results were supported by data indicating that resveratrol inhibited COX-2 promoter-dependent transcriptional activity and PKC activation [73].

7.3. EGCG and COX-2

Recent studies showed that EGCG significantly inhibited COX-2 and iNOS activity and nitric oxide production in LPS-activated Raw 264.7 cells [74], suggesting an effect mediated by NF-κB. However, not all COX-2 activation is associated directly with increased NF-κB activation and EGCG can also stimulate COX-2 expression. In the NMBA-induced rat esophageal tumorgenesis model, treatment with EGCG resulted in significantly less tumor development and tumor incidence. These results corresponded with decreased expression of cyclin D1 and COX-2 and decreased production of prostaglandin E2 [75]. Topical pre-treatment with green tea extract has been shown to block the acute COX-2 response to UVB in mice or humans [76]. Another recent study showed that pre-treatment of mice with EGCG significantly inhibited TPA-induced COX-2 expression in mouse skin and also in TPA-induced human mammary epithelial cells [77]. The inhibition was associated with a suppression of TPA-stimulated ERKs and p38 kinases activities, but surprisingly, had no effect on TPA-induced AP-1 DNA binding [80].

7.4. Ginger and COX-2

Gingerols have been shown to be effective inhibitors of arachidonic acid-induced platelet release and aggregation, an effect that was attributed to inhibition of

COX-2 [78]. Ginger components were also shown to inhibit COX-2 in cultured human airways epithelial A549 cells in a manner that was structure and dose-dependent [79]. Thus ginger may also act on COX-2 in addition to inducing apoptosis or inhibiting AP-1 activation.

8. Summary

CRC development is a multi-step process that lasts for 10 to 15 years. Thus, intestinal tumorgenesis provides us with the opportunity for early detection and even prevention.

Cancer prevention is certain to be a significant focus of research and intervention in the coming years, propelled by the realization that we will be able to identify both individuals susceptible to specific cancers, as well as the molecular targets that can alter or stop the carcinogenesis process.

Science and technology have evolved to a point where we are able to use our knowledge of cancer biology to identify individuals at risk and interrupt the process of malignant transformation at the level of the pre-cancerous lesion. Pharmacology and genetics are collaborating to develop new interventions for early detection, and novel chemoprevention agents designed to affect molecular targets linked to specific pre-malignant or predisposing conditions. Recent progress in these fields increases the likelihood that cancer can be prevented. However, the value of such prophylactic strategies has yet to be confirmed in the current ongoing randomized, double blind, placebo controlled studies.

In the intriguing jigsaw puzzle of cancer prevention, we now have a definite positive answer for the basic question "if", but several other parts of the equation (proper patient selection, ultimate drug, optimal dosage and duration) are missing. The most challenging task is to find the proper place for these interventions in the entire effort of cancer prevention, in subjects at risk for colorectal neoplasia, as well as in those at risk for other tumors. The achievement of this important goal may contribute to the conversion of CRC into a truly preventable disease, in up to 90% of cases.

COX-2 is now considered as a viable target for chemotherapy, especially since selective COX-2 inhibitors have improved safety profiles compared with nonselective NSAIDs and are much less toxic than most chemotherapeutic agents.

Nutritional or dietary factors have attracted a great deal of interest because of their perceived ability to act as highly effective chemopreventive agents. They are perceived as being generally safe and may have efficacy as chemopreventive agents by preventing or reversing premalignant lesions and/or reducing second primary tumor incidence. Many of these compounds appear to act on multiple tumors promoter-stimulated cellular pathways. Some of the most interesting and well documented are resveratrol and components of tea, EGCG, ginger and the aflavins. Other potentially effective dietary compounds include perillyl alcohol, PEITC and caffeine. Many of these compounds act by affecting multiple target signaling pathways including inducing apoptosis and/or suppressing AP-1, NF-κB and/or COX-2 expression, thus making them highly effective compounds for chemoprevention.

Curcumin may prove an important chemopreventive agent for colorectal and other types of cancers. Its usefulness in the chemoprevention of colon cancer can be further extended to patients developing colon cancer without mutations in the *APC* gene. Curcumin treatment decreases growth of colon cancer cells in through the COX-2 pathway or through the Wnt-signalling and the cell–cell adhesion pathways. Thus, the function of curcumin in intervening multi-cellular pathways with high-level safety and no toxicity makes it a wide-spectrum chemopreventive agent for colon cancer treatment.

Selective COX-2 inhibition has recently been investigated in various models of CRC in combination with inducible nitric oxide inhibitors [80], MMP inhibitors [81], ornithine decarboxylase inhibitors (difluoromethylornithine) [82] epidermal growth factor receptor kinase inhibitors [83,84] radiotherapy [85], and chemotherapy [86]. The majority of CRC over-express COX-2, and this increased expression is thought to inhibit apoptosis, induce angiogenesis, subvert the immune system, and promote tumor invasion. An understanding of the mechanism(s) whereby COX-2 mediates these phenomena awaits further studies.

The goal of future studies is to develop ways of blocking COX-2 activities without disrupting the cardiovascular system, since colorectal cancer is a common and deadly disease, and the potential benefit of primary prevention is great.

References

[1] M.H. Tattersall and H. Thomas, Recent advances: Oncology, *BMJ* **318** (1999), 445–448.

[2] A. Jemal, A. Thomas, T. Murray and M. Thun, Cancer statistics, *CA Cancer J Clin* **52** (2002), 23–47.

[3]	J. Walsh and J. Terdiman, CRCscreening, *JAMA* **289** (2003), 1288–1296.

[4]	B.W. Steward and P. Kleihues, eds, *World Cancer Report*, Lyon, IARC Press, 2003, 198–202.

[5]	M.R. Keighley, Gastrointestinal cancers in Europe, *Aliment Pharmacol Ther* **18** (2003), 7–30.

[6]	H.K. Weir, M.J. Thun, B.F. Hankey, L.A. Ries, H.L. Howe, P.A. Wingo, A. Jemal, E. Ward, R.N. Anderson and B.K. Edwards, Annual report to the nation on the status of cancer, 1975–2000, featuring the uses of surveillance data for cancer prevention and control, *J Natl Cancer Inst* **95** (2003), 1276–1299.

[7]	The International Agency for Research on Cancer (IARC), World Health Organization. http://www.iarc.fr/

[8]	W.K. Hong, S.M. Lippman, L.M. Itri, D.D. Karp, J.S. Lee, R.M. Byers, S.P. Schantz, A.M. Kramer, R. Lotan, L.J. Peters et al., Prevention of second primary tumors with isotretinoin in squamous-cell carcinoma of the head and neck, *N Engl J Med* **323** (1990), 795–801.

[9]	M.C. King, S. Wieand, K. Hale, M. Lee, T. Walsh, K. Owens, J. Tait, L. Ford, B.K. Dunn, J. Costantino, L. Wickerham, N. Wolmark and B. Fisher, National Surgical Adjuvant Breast and Bowel Project. Tamoxifen and breast cancer incidence among women with inherited mutations in BRCA1 and BRCA2: National Surgical Adjuvant Breast and Bowel Project (NSABP-P1) Breast Cancer Prevention Trial, *JAMA* **286** (2001), 2251–2256.

[10]	J. Cuzick, J. Forbes, R. Edwards, M. Baum, S. Cawthorn, A. Coates, A. Hamed, A. Howell and T. Powles, IBIS investigators.. First results from the International Breast Cancer Intervention Study (IBIS-I): a randomised prevention trial, *Lancet* **360** (2002), 817–824.

[11]	C.S. Williams, W. Smalley and R.N. DuBois, Aspirin use and potential mechanisms for CRCprevention, *J Clin Invest* **100** (1997), 1325 1329.

[12]	N. Arber, Do NSAIDs prevent colorectal cancer? *Can J Gastroenterol* **14** (2000), 299–307.

[13]	M. Moorghen, P. Ince, K.J. Finney, J.P. Sunter, D.R. Appleton and A.J. Watson, A protective effect of sulindac against chemically induced primary colonic tumours in mice, *J Pathol* **156** (1988), 341–347.

[14]	C.V. Rao, A. Rivenson, B. Simi, E. Zang, G. Kelloff, V. Steele and B.S. Reddy, Chemoprevention of colon carcinogenesis by sulindac, a nonsteroidal anti- inflammatory agent. *Cancer Res* **55** (1995), 1464–1472.

[15]	W.R. Waddell and R.W. Loughry, Sulindac for polyposis of the colon, *J Surg Oncol* **24** (1983), 83–87.

[16]	E. Giovannucci, K.M. Egan, D.J. Hunter, M.J. Stampfer, G.A. Colditz, W.C. Willett and F.E. Speizer, Aspirin and the risk of CRCin women, *N Engl J Med* **333** (1995), 609–614.

[17]	D. Loren, J. Lewis and M. Kochman, CRC: detection and prevention, *Gastroenterology clinics of North America* **31** (2002), 565–586.

[18]	L.M. Lichtenberger, Where is the evidence that cyclooxygenase inhibition is the primary cause of nonsteroidal anti-inflammatory drug (NSAID)-induced gastrointestinal injury? Topical injury revisited, *Biochem Pharmacol* **61** (2001), 631–637.

[19]	M.M. Wolfe, D.R. Lichtenstein and G. Singh, Gastrointestinal toxicity of nonsteroidal antiinflammatory drugs, *N Engl J Med* **340** (1999), 1888–1899.

[20]	M.M. Taketo, Cyclooxygenase-2 inhibitors in tumorigenesis, *J Natl Cancer Inst* **90** (1998), 1529–1536.

[21]	C.E. Eberhart, R.J. Coffey, A. Radhika, F.M. Giardiello, S. Ferrenbach and R.N. DuBois, Up regulation of cyclooxygenase 2 gene expression in human colorectal adenomas and adenocarcinomas, *Gastroenterology* **107** (1994), 1183–1188.

[22]	T. Fujita, M. Matsui, K. Takaku, H. Uetake, W. Ichikawa, M.M. Taketo and K. Sugihara, Size and invasion dependent increase in cyclooxygenase 2 levels in human colorectal carcinomas, *Cancer Res* **58** (1998), 4823–4826.

[23]	A.J. Dannenberg, N.K. Altorki, J.O. Boyle, C. Dang, L.R. Howe, B.B. Weksler and K. Subbaramaiah, Cyclo-oxygenase 2: A pharmacological target for the prevention of cancer, *Lancet Oncol* **2** (2001), 544–551.

[24]	W. Dempke, C. Rie, A. Grothey and H.J. Schmoll, Cyclooxygenase-2: A novel target for cancer chemotherapy? *J Cancer Res Clin Oncol* **127** (2001), 411–417.

[25]	E.R. Fearon and B. Vogelstein, A genetic model for colorectal tumorigenesis, *Cell* **61** (1990), 759–767.

[26]	C.E. Eberhart, R.J. Coffey, A. Radhika, F.M. Giardiello, S. Ferrenbach and R.N. DuBois, Up-regulation of cyclooxygenase 2 gene expression in human colorectal adenomas and adenocarcinomas, *Gastroenterology* **107** (1994), 1183–1188.

[27]	H. Sano, Y. Kawahito, R.L. Wilder, A. Hashiramoto, S. Mukai, K. Asai, S. Kimura, H. Kato, M. Kondo and T. Hla, Expression of cyclooxygenase-1 and -2 in human colorectal cancer, *Cancer Res* **55** (1995), 3785–3789.

[28]	D.A. Dixon, Regulation of COX-2 expression in human cancer, *Prog Exp Tumor Res* **37** (2003), 52–71.

[29]	S.L. Kargman, G.P. O'Neill, P.J. Vickers, J.F. Evans, J.A. Mancini and S. Jothy, Expression of prostaglandin G/H synthase-1 and -2 protein in human colon cancer, *Cancer Res* **55** (1995), 2556–2559.

[30]	C. Luong, A. Miller, J. Barnett, J. Chow, C. Ramesha and M.F. Browner, Flexibility of the NSAID binding site in the structure of human cyclooxygenase-2, *Nat Struct Biol* **3** (1996), 927–933.

[31]	R.G. Kurumbail, A.M. Stevens, J.K. Gierse, J.J. McDonald, R.A. Stegeman, J.Y. Pak, D. Gildehaus, J.M. Miyashiro, T.D. Penning, K. Seibert, P.C. Isakson and W.C. Stallings, Structural basis for selective inhibition of cyclooxygenase-2 by anti-inflammatory agents, *Nature* **384** (1996), 644–648.

[32]	D. Picot, P.J. Loll and R.M. Garavito, The x-ray crystal structure of the membrane protein prostaglandin H2 synthase-1, *Nature* **367** (1994), 243–249.

[33]	E. Wong, C. Bayly, H.L. Waterman, D. Riendeau and J.A. Mancini, Conversion of prostaglandin G/H synthase-1 into an enzyme sensitive to PGHS-2-selective inhibitors by a double His513 –> Arg and Ile523 –> val mutation, *J Biol Chem* **272** (1997), 9280–9286.

[34]	F.E. Silverstein, G. Faich, J.L. Goldstein, L.S. Simon, T. Pincus, A. Whelton, R. Makuch, G. Eisen, N.M. Agrawal, W.F. Stenson, A.M. Burr, W.W. Zhao, J.D. Kent, J.B. Lefkowith, K.M. Verburg and G.S. Geis, Gastrointestinal toxicity with celecoxib vs nonsteroidal anti-inflammatory drugs for osteoarthritis and rheumatoid arthritis: the CLASS study: A randomized controlled trial. Celecoxib Long-Term Arthritis Safety Study, *JAMA* **284** (2000), 1247–1255.

[35]	C. Bombardier, L. Laine, A. Reicin, D. Shapiro, R. Burgos-Vargas, B. Davis, R. Day, M.B. Ferraz, C.J. Hawkey, M.C. Hochberg, T.K. Kvien and T.J. Schnitzer, VIGOR Study Group. Comparison of upper gastrointestinal toxicity of rofecoxib and naproxen in patients with rheumatoid arthritis. VIGOR Study Group, *N Engl J Med* **343** (2000), 1520–1528, 2 p following 1528.

[36] S.D. Solomon, J.J. McMurray, M.A. Pfeffer, J. Wittes, R. Fowler, P. Finn, W.F. Anderson, A. Zauber, E. Hawk and M. Bertagnolli, Adenoma Prevention with Celecoxib (APC) Study Investigators. Cardiovascular risk associated with celecoxib in a clinical trial for colorectal adenoma prevention, *N Engl J Med* **352** (2005), 1071–1080.

[37] R.S. Bresalier, R.S. Sandler, H. Quan, J.A. Bolognese, B. Oxenius, K. Horgan et al., Cardiovascular events associated with rofecoxib in a colorectal adenoma chemoprevention trial, *N Engl J Med* **352** (2005), 1092–1102.

[38] M.M.E. Bertagnolli, CL and E.T. Hawk, Celecoxib reduces sporadic colorectal adenomas:result from the Adenoma Prevention with Celecoxib Trial, *Proc Am Assoc Cancer Res* **47** (2006), (Abstract CP-3).

[39] N. Arber, Chemoprevention of colorectal adenomas with celecoxib in an international randomized, placebo-controlled double-blind trial *Proc Am Assoc Cancer Res* **47** (2006), (Abstarct CP-4).

[40] N. Arber, C.J. Eagle, J. Spicak, I. Rácz, P. Dite, J. Hajer, M. Zavoral, M.J. Lechuga, P. Gerletti, J. Tang, R.B. Rosenstein, K. Macdonald, P. Bhadra, R. Fowler, J. Wittes, A.G. Zauber, S.D. Solomon and B. Levin, for the PreSAP Trial Investigators. Celecoxib for the Prevention of Colorectal Adenomatous Polyps, *N Engl J Med*, in press.

[41] T.A. Chan, P.J. Morin, B. Vogelstein and K.W. Kinzler, Mechanisms underlying nonsteroidal anti-inflammatory drug mediated apoptosis, *Proc Natl Acad Sci USA* **95** (1998), 681–686.

[42] M. Tsujii, S. Kawano, S. Tsuji, H. Sawaoka, M. Hori and R.N. DuBois, Cyclooxygenase regulates angiogenesis induced by colon cancer cells, *Cell* **93** (1998), 705–716.

[43] P. Janne and R. Mayer, Chemoprevention of colorectal cancer, *N Engl J Med* **342** (2000), 1960–1968.

[44] Y. Yamamoto, M.-J. Yin, K.-M. Lin and R.B. Gaynor, Sulindac inhibits activation of the NF-kappaB pathway, *J Biol Chem* **274** (1999), 27307–27314.

[45] T.-C. He, T.A. Chan, B. Vogelstein and K.W. Kinzler, PPARδ is an APC regulated target of nonsteroidal anti-inflammatory drugs, *Cell* **99** (1999), 335–345.

[46] S. Gately and R. Kerbel, Therapeutic potential of selective cyclooxygenase-2 inhibitors in the management of tumor angiogenesis, *Prog Exp Tumor Res* **37** (2003), 179–192.

[47] N. Chainani-Wu, Safety and anti-inflammatory activity of curcumin: A component of turmeric (*Curcuma longa*), *J Altern Complement Med* **9** (2003), 161–168.

[48] C.V. Rao, A. Rivenson, B. Simi and B.S. Reddy, Chemoprevention of colon carcinogenesis by dietary curcumin, a naturally occurring plant phenolic compound in mice, *Cancer Res* **55** (1995), 259–266.

[49] T. Kawamori, R. Lubet, V.E. Steele, G.J. Kelloff, R.B. Kaskey, C.V. Rao and B.S. Reddy, Chemopreventive effect of curcumin, a naturally occurring anti-inflammatory agent, during the promotion/progression stages of colon cancer, *Cancer Res* **59** (1999), 597–601.

[50] N.N. Mahmoud, A.M. Carothers, D. Grunberger, R.T. Bilinski, M.R. Churchill, C. Martucci, H.L. Newmark and M.M. Bertagnolli, Plant phenolics decrease intestinal tumours in an animal model of familial adenomatous polyposis, *Carcinogenesis* **21** (2000), 921–927.

[51] G.J. Kelloff, J.A. Crowell, E.T. Hawk, V.E. Steele, R.A. Lubet, C.W. Boone, J.M. Covey, L.A. Doody, G.S. Omenn, P. Greenwald, W.K. Hong, D.R. Parkinson, D. Bagheri, G.T. Baxter, M. Blunden, M.K. Doeltz, K.M. Eisenhauer, K. Johnson, G.G. Knapp, D.G. Longfellow, W.F. Malone, S.G. Nayfield, H.E. Seifried, L.M. Swallm and C.C. Sigman, Strategy and planning for chemopreventive drug development: Clinical development plans II, *J Cell Biochem* **26**(Suppl) (1996), 54–71.

[52] R.A. Sharma, H.R. McLelland, K.A. Hill, C.R. Ireson, S.A. Euden, M.M. Manson, M. Pirmohamed, L.J. Marnett, A.J. Gescher and W.P. Steward, Pharmacodynamic and pharmacokinetic study of oral Curcuma extract in patients with colorectal cancer, *Clin Cancer Res* **7** (2001), 1894–1900.

[53] A. Goel, C.R. Boland and D.P. Chauhan, Specific inhibition of cyclooxygenase-2 (COX-2) expression by dietary curcumin in HT-29 human colon cancer cells, *Cancer Lett* **172** (2001), 111–118.

[54] M. Sonoshita, K. Takaku, N. Sasaki, Y. Sugimoto, F. Ushikubi, S. Narumiya, M. Oshima and M.M. Taketo, Acceleration of intestinal polyposis through prostaglandin receptor EP2 in Apc(_716) knockout mice, *Nat Med* **7** (2001), 1048–1051.

[55] C. Williams, R.L. Shattuck-Brandt and R.N. DuBois, The role of COX-2 in intestinal cancer, *Ann NY Acad Sci* **889** (1999), 72–83.

[56] L. Korutla, J.Y. Cheung, J. Mendelsohn and R. Kumar, Inhibition of ligand-induced activation of epidermal growth factor receptor tyrosine phosphorylation by curcumin, *Carcinogenesis* **16** (1995), 1741–1745.

[57] M.C. Jiang, H.F. Yang-Yen, J.J. Yen and J.K. Lin, Curcumin induces apoptosis in immortalized NIH 3T3 and malignant cancer cell lines, *Nutr Cancer* **26** (1996), 111–120.

[58] S. Singh and B.B. Aggarwal, Activation of transcription factor NF-kappa B is suppressed by curcumin (diferuloylmethane), *J Biol Chem* **270** (1995), 24995–25000.

[59] S. Lev-Ari, L. Strier, D. Kazanov, L. Madar-Shapiro, H. Dvory-Sobol, I. Pinchuk, B. Marian, D. Lichtenberg and N. Arber, Curcumin potentiates the growth–inhibitory effect of celecoxib in human CRCcells, *Clin Can Res* (accepted) 2005.

[60] S. Lev-Ari, H. Zinger, D. Kazanov, D. Yona, E. Sagiv, S. Luria, R. BenYosef, A. Figer and N. Arber, Curcumin synergistically potentiates the growth-inhibitoryand pro-apoptotic effects of celecoxib in pancreatic adenocarcinoma cells, *Biomedicine & Pharmacotherapy* (accepted) 2005.

[61] J.E. Paulsen, I.K. Elvsaas, I.L. Steffensen and J. Alexander, A fish oil derived concentrate enriched in eicosapentaenoic and docosahexaenoic acid as ethyl ester suppresses the formation and growth of intestinal polyps in the Min mouse, *Carcinogenesis* **18** (1997), 1905–1910.

[62] M. Oshima, M. Takahashi, H. Oshima, M. Tsutsumi, K. Yazawa, T. Sugimura, S. Nishimura, K. Wakabayashi and M.M. Taketo, Effects of docosahexaenoic acid (DHA) on intestinal polyp development in Apc(Δ716) knockout mice, *Carcinogenesis* **16** (1995), 2605–2607.

[63] T.A. Chan, P.J. Morin, B. Vogelstein and K.W. Kinzler, Mechanisms underlying nonsteroidal antiinflammatory drug-mediated apoptosis, *Proc Natl Acad Sci USA* **95** (1998), 681–686.

[64] J.E. Paulsen, T. Stamm and J. Alexander, A fish oil-derived concentrate enriched in eicosapentaenoic and docosahexaenoic acid as ethyl esters inhibits the formation and growth of aberrant crypt foci in rat colon, *Pharmacol Toxicol* **82** (1998), 28–33.

[65] Y.J. Surh, K.S. Chun, H.H. Cha, S.S. Han, Y.S. Keum, K.K. Park and S.S. Lee, Molecular mechanisms underlying chemopreventive activities of anti-inflammatory phytochemicals: down-regulation of COX-2 and iNOS through suppression of NF-kappa B activation, *Mutat Res* **480–481** (2001), 243–268.

[66]   S.H. Tsai, Y.C. Liang, L. Chen, F.M. Ho, M.S. Hsieh and J.K. Lin, Arsenite stimulates cyclooxygenase-2 expression through activating IkappaB kinase and nuclear factor kappaB in primary and ECV304 endothelial cells, *J Cell Biochem* **84** (2002), 750–758.

[67]   S.R. Adderley and D.J. Fitzgerald, Oxidative damage of cardiomyocytes is limited by extracellular regulated kinases 1/2-mediated induction of cyclooxygenase-2, *J Biol Chem* **274** (1999), 5038–5046.

[68]   H.Q. Wang, M.P. Kim, H.F. Tiano, R. Langenbach and R.C. Smart, Protein kinase C-alpha coordinately regulates cytosolic phospholipase A(2) activity and the expression of cyclooxygenase-2 through different mechanisms in mouse keratinocytes, *Mol Pharmacol* **59** (2001), 860–866.

[69]   H. Niiro, T. Otsuka, E. Ogami, K. Yamaoka, S. Nagano, M. Akahoshi, H. Nakashima, Y. Arinobu, K. Izuhara and Y. Niho, MAP kinase pathways as a route for regulatory mechanisms of IL-10 and IL-4 which inhibit COX-2 expression in human monocytes, *Biochem Biophys Res Commun* **250** (1998), 200–205.

[70]   M. Jang, L. Cai, G.O. Udeani, K.V. Slowing, C.F. Thomas, C.W. Beecher, H.H. Fong, N.R. Farnsworth, A.D. Kinghorn, R.G. Mehta, R.C. Moon and J.M. Pezzuto, Cancer chemopreventive activity of resveratrol, a natural product derived from grapes, *Science* **275** (1997), 218–220.

[71]   Z.G. Li, T. Hong, Y. Shimada, I. Komoto, A. Kawabe, Y. Ding, J. Kaganoi, Y. Hashimoto and M. Imamura, Suppression of *N*-nitrosomethylbenzylamine (NMBA)-induced esophageal tumorigenesis in F344 rats by resveratrol, *Carcinogenesis* **23** (2002), 1531–1536.

[72]   K. Subbaramaiah, W.J. Chung, P. Michaluart, N. Telang, T. Tanabe, H. Inoue, M. Jang, J.M. Pezzuto and A.J. Dannenberg, Resveratrol inhibits cyclooxygenase-2 transcription and activity in phorbol ester-treated human mammary epithelial cells, *J Biol Chem* **273** (1998), 21875–21882.

[73]   J. Garcia-Garcia, V. Micol, A. de Godos and J.C. Gomez-Fernandez, The cancer chemopreventive agent resveratrol is incorporated into model membranes and inhibits protein kinase C alpha activity, *Arch Biochem Biophys* **372** (1999), 382–388.

[74]   S.J. Lee, I.S. Lee and W. Mar, Inhibition of inducible nitric oxide synthase and cyclooxygenase-2 activity by 1,2,3,4,6-penta-O-galloyl-beta-D-glucose in murine macrophage cells, *Arch Pharm Res* **26** (2003), 832–839.

[75]   Z.G. Li, Y. Shimada, F. Sato, M. Maeda, A. Itami, J. Kaganoi, I. Komoto, A. Kawabe and M. Imamura, Inhibitory effects of epigallocatechin-3-gallate on N-nitrosomethylbenzylamine-induced esophageal tumorigenesis in F344 rats, *Int J Oncol* **21** (2002), 1275–1283.

[76]   K.P. An, M. Athar, X. Tang, S.K. Katiyar, J. Russo, J. Beech, M. Aszterbaum, L. Kopelovich, E.H. Epstein Jr., H. Mukhtar and D.R. Bickers, Cyclooxygenase-2 expression in murine and human non-melanoma skin cancers: implications for therapeutic approaches, *Photochem Photobiol* **76** (2002), 73–80.

[77]   J.K. Kundu, H.K. Na, K.S. Chun, Y.K. Kim, S.J. Lee, S.S. Lee, O.S. Lee, Y.C. Sim and Y.J. Surh, Inhibition of phorbol ester-induced COX-2 expression by epigallocatechin gallate in mouse skin and cultured human mammary epithelial cells, *J Nutr* **133** (2003), 3805S–3810S.

[78]   K.L. Koo, A.J. Ammit, V.H. Tran, C.C. Duke and B.D. Roufogalis, Gingerols and related analogues inhibit arachidonic acid-induced human platelet serotonin release and aggregation, *Thromb Res* **103** (2001), 387–397.

[79]   E. Tjendraputra, V.H. Tran, D. Liu-Brennan, B.D. Roufogalis and C.C. Duke, Effect of ginger constituents and synthetic analogues on cyclooxygenase-2 enzyme in intact cells, *Bioorg Chem* **29** (2001), 156–163.

[80]   C.V. Rao, C. Indranie, B. Simi, P.T. Manning, J.R. Connor and B.S. Reddy, Chemopreventive properties of a selective inducible nitric oxide synthase inhibitor in colon carcinogenesis, administered alone or in combination with celecoxib, a selective cyclooxygenase-2 inhibitor, *Cancer Res* **62** (2002), 165–170.

[81]   R.A. Wagenaar-Miller, G. Hanley, R. Shattuck-Brandt, R.N. DuBois, R.L. Bell, L.M. Matrisian and D.W. Morgan, Cooperative effects of matrix metalloproteinase and cyclooxygenase-2 inhibition on intestinal adenoma reduction, *Br J Cancer* **88** (2003), 1445–1452.

[82]   S.M. Fischer, C.J. Conti, J. Viner, C.M. Aldaz and R.A. Lubet, Celecoxib and difluoromethylornithine in combination have strong therapeutic activity against UV-induced skin tumors in mice, *Carcinogenesis* **24** (2003), 945–952.

[83]   C.J. Torrance, P.E. Jackson, E. Montgomery, K.W. Kinzler, B. Vogelstein, A. Wissner, M. Nunes, P. Frost and C.M. Discafani, Combinatorial chemoprevention of intestinal neoplasia, *Nat Med* **6** (2000), 1024–1028.

[84]   M. Mann, H. Sheng, J. Shao, C.S. Williams, P.I. Pisacane, M.X. Sliwkowski and R.N. DuBois, Targeting cyclooxygenase 2 and HER-2/neu pathways inhibits colorectal carcinoma growth, *Gastroenterology* **120** (2001), 1713–1719.

[85]   A.P. Dicker, T.L. Williams and D.S. Grant, Targeting angiogenic processes by combination rofecoxib and ionizing radiation, *Am J Clin Oncol* **24** (2001), 438–442.

[86]   M. Yao, S. Kargman, E.C. Lam, C.R. Kelly, P. Luk, E. Kwong, J.F. Evans and M.M. Wolfe, Inhibition of cyclooxygenase-2 by rofecoxib attenuates the growth and metastatic potential of colorectal carcinoma in mice, *Cancer Res* **63** (2003), 586–592.

Cancer Biomarkers 3 (2007) 163–168
IOS Press

Genetic testing to identify high-risk populations for chemoprevention studies

Jonathan L. Velasquez* and Steven M. Lipkin
*Departments of Medicine, Divisions of Hematology-Oncology and Epidemiology, University of California, 839
Medical Sciences Court, 2nd Floor, Sprague Hall – Lab 250, Irvine, CA 92697, USA*

Abstract. Human genetic variation data is now publicly available on a large scale, from both public and private discovery efforts. Datasets from the International Haplotype Map Consortium and Perlegen Sciences provide a level of knowledge about human genetic variation that is unprecedented. In combination with novel high-throughput genotyping technologies, these new resources will allow cancer prevention investigators to identify in a more precise way which genetic subsets of patients are likely to benefit most from chemoprevention and screening interventions.

Keywords: SNPs, haplotypes, chemoprevention

1. Introduction

Many genes that contribute to highly penetrant cancer risk have been discovered using an approach that takes advantage of highly informative families with many affected relatives and a well characterized phenotype. Whole genome linkage analysis has been the most successful strategy to identify rare, highly penetrant genes relevant to cancer. Their identification has allowed intensive early detection surveillance strategies to prevent cancer and improve survival [15]. Newer strategies such as sib-pair studies have recently identified candidate regions of interest and are likely to yield contributing genes as well, but these approaches often have difficulties mapping genetic intervals down to the resolution necessary for disease gene identification [28]. Genotyping technology has recently evolved to increase the resolution of genome scans by several orders of magnitude. Genetic association studies have greater statistical power to exploit the more recent high-throughput genotyping methods. They can measure how genetic variation contributes to cause specific individuals to be at high risk of malignancy. In the near future we will see important studies that go beyond the characterization of rare highly penetrant genetic syndromes, and which will yield important insights about how genetic variation influences clinical response to specific cancer chemoprevention agents for sporadic cancer.

2. What are SNPs?

Single Nucleotide Polymorphisms (SNPs; pronounced "snips") are the most common known form of human genetic variation, and estimated to account for greater than 90% of total human genetic variation [3,12]. The genomic variation existing today among mankind is the result of $\sim$50,000–100,000 years of evolution of many different genomic and population events, with evolutionary selection occurring with punctuated equilibrium (such as hypothesized to occur during the last Ice Age $\sim$20,000 years ago). Most of this variation has no obvious pathological medical significance. Polymorphisms are distinguished from mutations by an arbitrary frequency criterion: The different forms of the polymorphism (termed "alleles") are observed more often in the general population than mutations, with a population frequency of $<1\%$ often used as a cutoff value [4,5]. SNPs almost always have

*Corresponding author. Tel.: +1 949 824 9221; Fax: +1 949 824 4405; E-mail: jvelasqu@uci.edu, slipkin@uci.edu.

a major (more frequent) and minor (less frequent) allele. These are caused by a substitution of one base for another. The most common type of SNP are transitions: purines are replaced by purines and pyrimidines by pyrimidines (e.g., C to T or A to G). Because humans are diploid for each SNP a person can have one of several genotypes: homozygous for the major allele, heterozygous, or homozygous for the minor allele (e.g. AA, Aa or aa). Five-methyl cytosine is the most common modified DNA base residue. Because 5-methyl cytosine can be spontaneously converted to thymine, C to T SNPs are the most common in the human genome (4).

3. What are haplotypes?

Sets of single nucleotide polymorphisms (SNPs) can be genotyped across a genomic segment to characterize the specific chromosomes that exist in a population; the combination of alleles that exist along a chromosome is termed a haplotype. Haplotypes are a combination of alleles at different markers along the same chromosome that are inherited as a unit [3,4] (Fig. 1). The fundamental difference between haplotypes and individual genotypes at SNPs is that the alleles are assigned to a chromosome. In essence, each individual has two haplotypes for a given stretch of the genome, representing the maternal and paternal chromosomes. In practice, haplotypes provide increased statistical power to detect association and map etiological mutations over classical single-marker approaches, as well as greatly reducing the amount of genotyping required to evaluate the role of common genetic variation on a clinical outcome.

4. Chemoprevention and genetically defined patient subsets

It has long been recognized that the same medications cause different responses in different patients. Large differences in drug response between human populations, combined with small intra-patient variability, suggest a genetic contribution to drug disposition and effects with estimates ranging from 20–90% [9]. Genetic variation in both drug targets and genes affecting target signal transduction can have a profound effect on drug efficacy and toxicity, with $\geqslant 25$ known examples [9]. These include variants in genes relevant both therapeutics and prevention.

Gene variation and haplotypes associated with , antineoplastic therapeutics such as Rituxan [27], thiopurines (TPMT) [8], irinotecan and gemcitabine among others [10,16–18] have been extensively studied. Cancer chemoprevention has identified specific pharmacologic and/or dietary agents that decrease incidence of specific cancers. Perhaps the best known examples are that of aspirin and other non-steroidal antiinflammatory agents (NSAIDs) in colorectal cancer (CRC) prevention. In terms of CRC, this area has been extensively characterized in the high-penetrance genetic CRC syndromes. Because the progression from initiation of adenoma to carcinoma can take several years, prevention can have a major impact on morbidity and mortality. NSAIDs and the more selective cycloxygenase-2 (COX-2) inhibitors have demonstrated significant chemopreventative benefits in Familial Adenomatous Polyposis (FAP). Four multi-arm randomized, placebo controlled trials have demonstrated that sulindac and celecoxib significantly reduce both the number and size of rectal adenomas in FAP patients (for recent review, see [13]). When combined, these data suggest the benefits for 4–6 months of sulindac causes a ~70% drop in the rectal adenoma rate, and ~25% drop in patients treated with Celecoxib. There are currently several ongoing chemoprevention trials for HNPCC. There is a celecoxib study that is a randomized, placebo-controlled Phase I/II multi-center trial evaluating the safety and efficacy of celecoxib in HNPCC [1]. The effects of these treatment arms on a number of endoscopic and tissue-based biomarker endpoints will be evaluated at baseline and 12 months. The CAPP2 study (Concerted Action Polyp Prevention) evaluates the preventative effects of aspirin and resistant starch in HNPCC carriers. In this study, carriers of HNPCC are randomized to received enteric coated aspirin or placebo combined with either starch or placebo (4 armed trial). The primary endpoint of the study will be the number, size, and histological stage of CRC found after 2 years on treatment or placebo [1]. In summary, these studies demonstrate the benefit of chemoprevention in a genetically defined group of patients with highly penetrant disease susceptibility. In the next generation, it is anticipated that more precisely defined subsets of patients suffering from "sporadic" cancer can be identified by haplotypes.

5. HMG CoA reductase inhibitors and cancer prevention

Recently, it has been discovered that HMG CoA-Reductase inhibitors ("statins" such as atovarstatin,

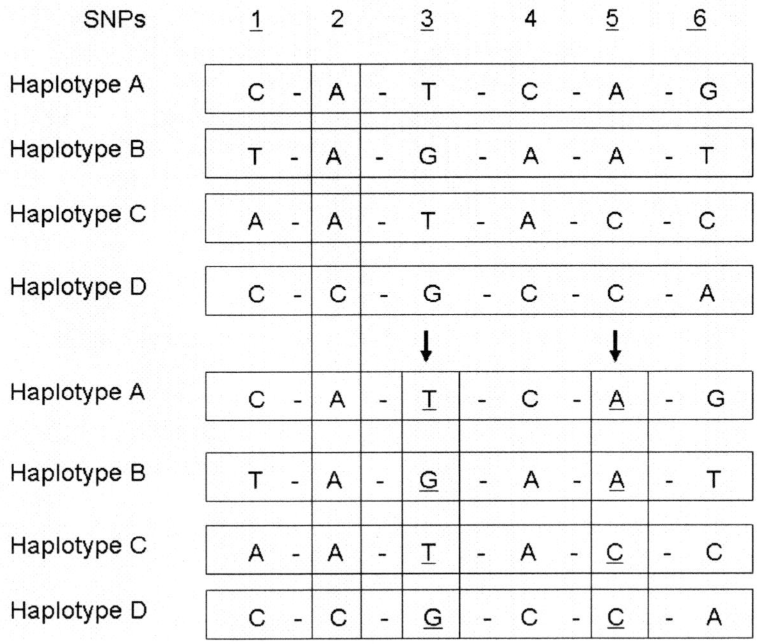

	SNPs	1	2	3	4	5	6
Haplotype A		C -	A -	T -	C -	A -	G
Haplotype B		T -	A -	G -	A -	A -	T
Haplotype C		A -	A -	T -	A -	C -	C
Haplotype D		C -	C -	G -	C -	C -	A
Haplotype A		C -	A -	T -	C -	A -	G
Haplotype B		T -	A -	G -	A -	A -	T
Haplotype C		A -	A -	T -	A -	C -	C
Haplotype D		C -	C -	G -	C -	C -	A

Fig. 1. Schematic representation of haplotype tag SNPs. A small hypothetical gene is diagrammed, in which there are six SNPs with moderately strong Linkage Disequilibrium (LD). Four of the six SNPs are known and in the public databases (annotated as underlined numbers), two are observed from genotyping subjects in chemoprevention studies, and one of these causes an increased chemoprevention efficacy for colorectal cancer. These four known SNPs have been genotyped by the HapMap project. In this particular population, only four combinations of alleles, or haplotypes (A, B, C, and D), account for all the diversity among the individuals. Suppose that one allele of SNP 2 (the minor variant G allele) increases the chemoprevention efficacy for colorectal cancer. In the upper panel, all six SNPs are diagrammed. SNPs 1, 3, 5, and 6 have been genotyped by the HapMap and used to define haplotypes A-D. SNPs 2 and 4 are SNPs whose alleles are located on those haplotypes. The long vertical box highlights the position of the disease-associated variant (the G allele of SNP 2). Genotyping of all four known SNPs (SNP 1, 3, 5, and 6) will allow for the testing of each individual haplotype for association with increased chemoprevention efficacy for colorectal cancer. Association between haplotype D and chemopreventative efficacy with reference to colorectal cancer will be detected, identifying it as the risk haplotype, although not identifying which SNP(s) is causing the association. In the lower panel, the same information can be obtained more efficiently by testing the htSNPs, SNP 3 and 5 (highlighted by the short boxes and arrows). Follow-up studies are then required to identify all SNPs that are present on the risk haplotype, as well as biological experiments, to correctly identify SNP 2 as the causative SNP. SNP, single nucleotide polymorphism; LD, linkage disequilibrium; htSNP, haplotype tagging single nucleotide polymorphism. After Sklar. (Sklar 2005).

pravachol or simvastatin) whose primary indication is cardiovascular disease prevention have significant chemoprevention activity in multiple cancers, but most impressively in colorectal cancer [11,21]. While the statins have been extensively studied in clinical trials assessing cardiovascular risk, most studies have not had either long-term follow up or the appropriate institutional approvals to link to CRC related outcomes. However, this endpoint was assessed in the Cholesterol and Recurrent Events (CARE) trial. This trial was designed primarily to evaluate the long-term effects of pravastatin on plasma concentration of C-reactive protein. They observed a significant reduction in CRC risk in pravastatin users vs. the placebo group (O.R. = 0.57). This observation has been become more intriguing with the subsequent association of elevated CRP levels with elevated CRC risk [7]. However, the relatively small number of CRC events in the CARE trial has made drawing conclusions about this relationship difficult. Graaf et al. recently conducted a large-scale retrospective study of statin use and risk of all types of cancer. Using the PHARMO database from the Netherlands, they identified more than 3,000 statin users from pharmacy records and almost 17,000 matched controls. Their data suggested that statins are protective when used longer than 4 years (adjusted OR, 0.64; 95% CI), although there was no breakdown available by individual types of cancer [11]. Recently, robust new data were presented supporting a role for statin drugs in CRC prevention [21]. The hypothesis that statin use is associated with CRC prevention was tested directly in this large study (1814 CRC cases and 1959 control subjects) of the Israeli population-based Molecular Epidemiology of Colon Cancer cohort [15,21]. Medication history was confirmed by personal interviews, and 96.5% of reported statin use was confirmed by prescription records with the Israeli Health Service records. Odds ratios were used to estimate relative risk and logistic regression used to adjust for other risk factors. Comparing subjects using statins for >5 years to non-users, overall a 51% relative risk reduction was observed for CRC (OR = 0.49 95% CI, 0.38–0.62; $p < 0.0001$) [21]. When adjusted for possible confounding factors between case and control subject groups of Aspirin/NSAID use, ethnicity, family history of CRC, physical activity, dietary vegetable intake and hypercholesterolemia, the adjusted OR was 0.54 (95% CI 0.39–0.75; $p < 0.0001$). Similar results were seen when subsets were separately analyzed for colon (OR = 0.53 95% CI 0.36–0.76 $p < 0.0007$) and rectal (OR = 0.38 95% CI 0.19–0.73; $p < 0.0038$) cancers, suggesting the effects of statins are not GI-tract location-specific and share mechanisms common to both anatomical sites. Similar risk reduction profiles were observed when analyzed separately for Pravastatin (OR = 0.45 95% CI 0.31–0.64; $p < 0.0001$) or Simvastatin (OR = 0.47 95% CI 0.34–0.65; $p < 0.0001$) users (Odds Ratio = 1.0 95% CI 0.55–1.93; $p = 0.936$, suggesting the chemopreventive effects are not "brand specific." No evidence of synergy between Statins and Aspirin/NSAIDs was observed ($p = 0.54$).

The contribution of human genetic variation to sporadic cancer chemoprevention is poorly defined at this point in time. It is well appreciated that human pharmacologic response to NSAID treatment is highly variable. In terms of cardiovascular risk prevention, it is striking that 25% of individuals taking aspirin do not respond by increased bleeding time or other significant aspects of platelet dysfunction in clotting [23]. Like aspirin, in clinical users of HMG coA reductase inhibitor/statin drugs for cardiovascular risk reduction, there is wide variation in inter-individual response to statin therapy. It has been hypothesized that genetic differences significantly contribute to this variation [2, 6,20,22,26]. Recently, with reference to the use of genetic screening to guide lipid-lowering therapy, genetic analyses of 1536 subjects from the PRINCE cardiovascular risk reduction clinical trial were used to test the hypothesis that common genetic variants influence the degree of lipid level reduction during pravastatin therapy [2]. Studying a number of cholesterol synthesis and transport candidate genes, genetic variation was examined for associations with changes in lipid levels during pravastatin therapy. Two tightly linked single nucleotide polymorphisms (SNPs) occurring in a haplotype from the *HMGCR* gene were identified as-

sociated with a 22% reduction in pravastatin therapy lipid lowering efficacy ($P < 0.001$) [2]. Interestingly, the SNPs in this haplotype did not affect lipid levels in a second group of 649 subjects who did not receive pravastatin therapy [2]. Non-statistically significant trends were also found for SNPs in the *squalene synthase* and *cholesteryl ester transfer protein* genes [2]. The investigators concluded that the cholesterol synthesis genetic variants identified in their study are likely to contribute significantly to impaired lipid lowering responses in treated subjects.

6. The application of SNPs and haplotypes to cancer chemoprevention

Can SNPs and haplotypes be applied to chemoprevention for sporadic cancer beyond the high penetrance syndromes? The authors are hopeful that we will see significant progress in the coming years. The ability to identify genetic markers associated with cancer prevention has greatly advanced in recent years. High-throughput technologies have also evolved, and now allow economical and rapid large-scale genotyping of large patient groups in therapeutic clinical trials. The HapMap and Perlegen initiatives have identified sets of SNPs that will characterize the common haplotypes across the human genome in the major ethnic groups. This initiative, combined with other public efforts to identify SNPs across specific gene regions, will greatly reduce the amount of genotyping required for genome-wide or candidate gene association studies of clinical phenotypes including cancer prevention and drug response.

The technology and bioinformatic resources for first generation Whole Genome Association (WGA) studies to identify genes important for important phenotypes such as clinical response to specific chemoprevention agents for cancer have arrived. The technical aspects of genotyping are now in place, the statistical methods have been developed and implemented in other studies. Recently a large-scale, case-control study successfully identified at least one susceptibility gene to a complex genetic trait, yet this study of myocardial infarction provides an important background for the whole genome study of chemoprevention responses. In a study of 1,133 cases and 1,006 controls, Ozaki et al. identified a gene on 6p21 associated with susceptibility to myocardial infarction [19]. The authors studied 92,788 SNPs, and 65,671(70.8%) of these SNPs could be successfully genotyped. Using a high-throughput genotyping strategy permitted them to screen 13,738 genes. One of these genes, lymphotoxin-α (*LTA*), was associated with an increased risk of myocardial infarction, odds ratio $= 1.78$, $p = 0.00000033$. This association was validated in a replication dataset with careful control for population stratification. Functional studies identified two SNPs with recognizable mechanisms, one of which induces a cell adhesion molecule expressed in vascular smooth muscle cells of human coronary arteries, and the other that leads to increased expression of *LTA*. Although whole genome association studies for cancer prevention have not yet been completed (as far as we are aware), the technical aspects of genotyping are now in place, the statistical methods have been developed and implemented in other studies, and existing specimens from clinical trial resources are well-positioned to take advantage of this approach to better understand genetic contributions to both cancer prevention and therapeutic response. There are currently at least 6 ongoing Whole Genome Association studies. (1) Whole Genome Association Study of HDL Level Modifiers (PI Kelly Frazer, Pfizer, New York, NY). (2). Colorectal Cancer (PI Stephen B. Gruber, University of Michigan, Ann Arbor, Michigan), (3) Autism (PI Aravinda Chakravarti, Johns Hopkins University, Baltimore, MD), (4) Alzheimer Disease (PI Jeff Trent, Translational Genomics Institute, Phoenix, AZ). (5) Swedish and American Type II Diabetes Determinants (PI David Altschuler, Broad Institute, Cambridge MA) and (6) Whole Genome Association Scan for Type II Diabetes in the Finnish Population (PI Francis Collins, NHGRI, Bethesda, MD). Three of these studies (1,2 and 6) utilize Perlegen WGA scanning technology, two (3, and 5) use Illumina BeadArray technology, and one (4) uses Affymtrix High Density 500K SNP Mapping Chips. (N.B. The specific pros and cons of each technology are beyond the scope of the discussion for this Review).

7. Conclusions

In summary, it is clear that human pharmacologic response to NSAIDs, statins and other well established active cancer chemoprevention agents is highly variable, and that much of this variation is attributable to genetic factors [25]. A new generation of mapping tools and technologies has been developed that exploit recent advances in our knowledge of the roles that SNPs and haplotypes. These advances allow an unprecedented level of precision to map the contribution of genetic factors to cancer chemoprevention. Using the examples of

NSAID and statin chemoprevention of CRC as a model, there are both ongoing and completed large scale clinical trials in which it is anticipated that genetic stratification can help identify patient subpopulations demonstrating clinical benefits that might otherwise be diluted and not recognized in a group of heterogeneous admixed cancer subtypes with different biological causes. The inclusion of genetic stratification is likely to help identify a high-risk patient population at increased cancer risk who are especially likely to benefit from statin or NSAID chemoprevention. Furthermore, because of recent requests by the US Food and Drug Administration to accept pharmacogenetic data in new drug applications, SNPs and haplotypes provide the underlying biological rationale for genetically stratified secondary endpoint analyses of chemoprevention trials that fail to demonstrate statistically significant benefit in the entire intent-to-treat trial population.

References

[1]   H.J. Annie Yu, K.M. Lin et al., Hereditary nonpolyposis colorectal cancer: preventive management, *Cancer Treat Rev* **29**(6) (2003), 461–470.

[2]   D.I. Chasman, D. Posada et al., Pharmacogenetic study of statin therapy and cholesterol reduction, *Jama* **291**(23) (2004), 2821–2827.

[3]   F.S. Collins, Genome research: the next generation, *Cold Spring Harb Symp Quant Biol* **68** (2003), 49–54.

[4]   D.C. Crawford, D.T. Akey et al., The Patterns of Natural Variation in Human Genes, *Annu Rev Genomics Hum Genet* (2005).

[5]   D.C. Crawford and D.A. Nickerson, Definition and clinical importance of haplotypes, *Annu Rev Med* **56** (2005), 303–320.

[6]   E. De Groot, J.W. Jukema et al., Effect of pravastatin on progression and regression of coronary atherosclerosis and vessel wall changes in carotid and femoral arteries: a report from the Regression Growth Evaluation Statin Study, *Am J Cardiol* **76**(9) (1995), 40C–46C.

[7]   T.P. Erlinger, E.A. Platz et al., C-reactive protein and the risk of incident colorectal cancer, *Jama* **291**(5) (2004), 585–590.

[8]   W.E. Evans, Pharmacogenetics of thiopurine S-methyltransferase and thiopurine therapy, *Ther Drug Monit* **26**(2) (2004), 186–191.

[9]   W.E. Evans and H.L. McLeod, Pharmacogenomics–drug disposition, drug targets, and side effects, *N Engl J Med* **348**(6) (2003), 538–549.

[10] A.K. Fukunaga, S. Marsh et al., Identification and analysis of single-nucleotide polymorphisms in the gemcitabine pharmacologic pathway, *Pharmacogenomics J* **4**(5) (2004), 307–314.

[11] M.R. Graaf, A.B. Beiderbeck et al., The risk of cancer in users of statins, *J Clin Oncol* **22**(12) (2004), 2388–2394.

[12] D.A. Hinds, L.L. Stuve et al., Whole-genome patterns of common DNA variation in three human populations, *Science* **307**(5712) (2005), 1072–1079.

[13] J.J. Keller and F.M. Giardiello, Chemoprevention strategies using NSAIDs and COX-2 inhibitors, *Cancer Biol Ther* **2**(4 Suppl 1) (2003), S140–149.

[14] S.M. Lipkin, L.S. Rozek et al., The MLH1 D132H variant is associated with susceptibility to sporadic colorectal cancer, *Nat Genet* **36**(7) (2004), 694–699.

[15] H.T. Lynch, B.D. Riley et al., Hereditary nonpolyposis colorectal carcinoma (HNPCC) and HNPCC-like families: Problems in diagnosis, surveillance, and management, *Cancer* **100**(1) (2004), 53–64.

[16] S. Marsh and H.L. McLeod, Cancer pharmacogenetics, *Br J Cancer* **90**(1) (2004), 8–11.

[17] S. Marsh and H.L. McLeod, Pharmacogenetics of irinotecan toxicity, *Pharmacogenomics* **5**(7) (2004), 835–843.

[18] H.L. McLeod, C.R. King et al., Application of pharmacogenomics in the individualization of chemotherapy for gastrointestinal malignancies, *Clin Colorectal Cancer* **4**(Suppl 1) (2004), S43–47.

[19] K. Ozaki, Y. Ohnishi et al., Functional SNPs in the lymphotoxin-alpha gene that are associated with susceptibility to myocardial infarction, *Nat Genet* **32**(4) (2002), 650–654.

[20] C. Packham, J. Robinson et al., Statin prescribing in Nottingham general practices: a cross-sectional study, *J Public Health Med* **21**(1) (1990), 60–64.

[21] J.N. Poynter, S.B. Gruber et al., Statins and the risk of colorectal cancer, *N Engl J Med* **352**(21) (2005), 2184–2192.

[22] L. Puccetti, A.L. Pasqui et al., Time-dependent effect of statins on platelet function in hypercholesterolaemia, *Eur J Clin Invest* **32**(12) (2002), 901–908.

[23] G. Siest, E. Jeannesson et al., Pharmacogenomics and drug response in cardiovascular disorders, *Pharmacogenomics* **5**(7) (2004), 779–802.

[24] P. Sklar, Principles of haplotype mapping and potential applications to attention-deficit/hyperactivity disorder, *Biol Psychiatry* **57**(11) (2005), 1357–1366.

[25] S.D. Undevia, G. Gomez-Abuin et al., Pharmacokinetic variability of anticancer agents, *Nat Rev Cancer* **5**(6) (2005), 447–458.

[26] B.A. Van Hout and M.L. Simoons, Cost-effectiveness of HMG coenzyme reductase inhibitors; whom to treat? *Eur Heart J* **22**(9) (2001), 751–761.

[27] W.K. Weng and R. Levy, Two immunoglobulin G fragment C receptor polymorphisms independently predict response to rituximab in patients with follicular lymphoma, *J Clin Oncol* **21**(21) (2003), 3940–3947.

[28] G.L. Wiesner, D. Daley et al., A subset of familial colorectal neoplasia kindreds linked to chromosome 9q22.2–31.2, *Proc Natl Acad Sci USA* **100**(22) (2003), 12961–12965.

Biomarkers in Drug Development
12th – 13th September 2007 London, UK

MAXIMISING APPLICATIONS OF BIOMARKERS WITHIN DEVELOPMENT

ACI's Biomarkers in Drug Development Conference will address the latest applications of biomarkers within drug discovery and development, with a key focus on integrating biomarkers earlier in clinical development, and maximising their use as part of a personalised approach to treatment.

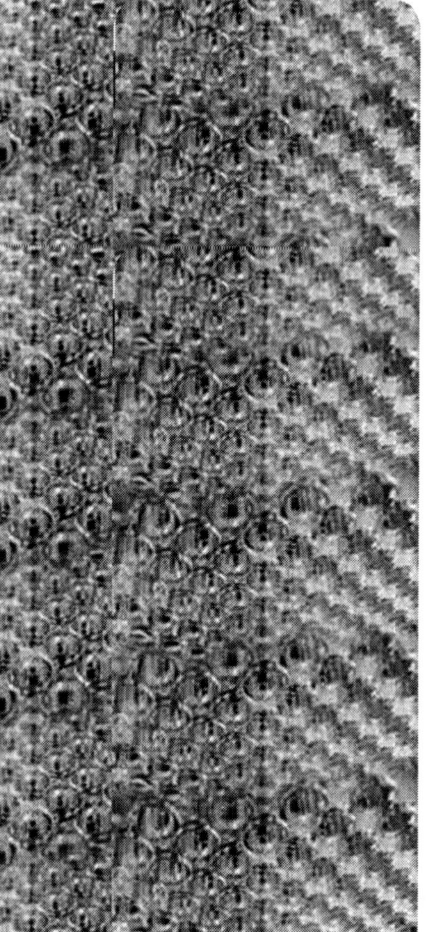

THE PROGRAMME WILL FOCUS ON KEY TOPICS INCLUDING:

- Biomarkers in early safety and toxicity assessment
- Biomarkers as validation tools – determining validation parameters
- Challenges in development and implementation of biomarkers
- Integrating biomarkers earlier – using markers in early clinical development
- Translational biomarkers – bridging the gap
- Biomarkers as companion in vitro diagnostics
- Using Biomarkers to stratify treatments applications

AMONG THE SPEAKERS:

- **Dr. Andrew Lockhart,** CPDM-Neurology Biomarker Group, GlaxoSmithKline
- **Dr. Ann Kapoun,** Associate Director, Biomarker R&D, Clinical Pharmacology & Experimental Medicine, ALZA
- **Dr. Eric Blomme,** Project Leader, Cell and Molecular Toxicology, Abbott Laboratories
- **Dr. Birgitte Soegaard,** Head, Clinical Pharmacology & Pharmacokinetics, H. Lundbeck A/S
- **Dr. Brian Swanson,** US Head of Biomarkers, Clinical and Experimental Pharmacology, Sanofi-Aventis

WHO WILL ATTEND?

Attendees will be drawn from pharmaceutical and biotechnology companies, and will include VPs, Directors and Managers of: Biomarkers, Translational/Experimental Medicine, Clinical Research/Development, Pharmacology, Toxicology and Safety Assessment, Clinical PK/PD, Discovery Medicine, Molecular Medicine/Diagnostics

REGISTRATION AND INFORMATION

The spaces at the event are very limited.
Therefore we always advise a quick registration.

To reserve your space or get additional information contact **Melanie Mulazzi on +44 207 368 1654 or email mmulazzi@acius.net**

SUPPORTING ORGANISATIONS

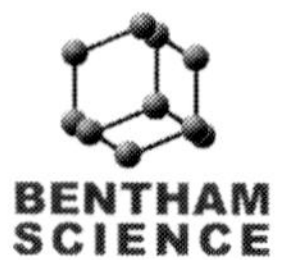
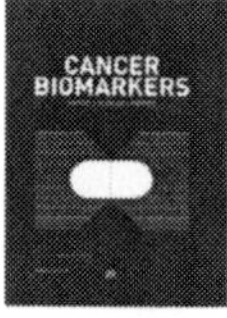
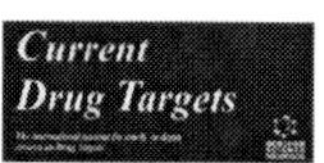
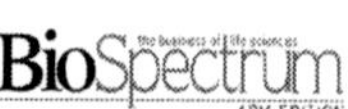
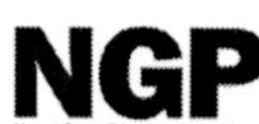
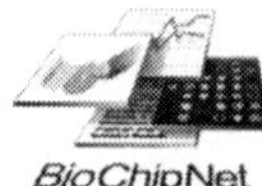
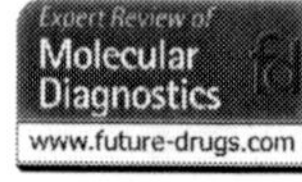
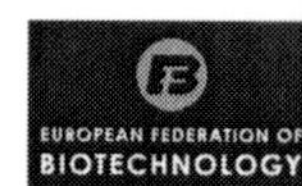

ACI's FORTHCOMING PHARMACEUTICAL EVENTS INCLUDE:

Vaccine Research and Development September 2007   **Drug Delivery Systems** October 2007
Molecular Diagnostics November 2007   **Imaging in Clinical Trials** January 2008
Antibodies in Discovery and Developments March 2008

Active Communications Europe Ltd • Tel: 0(+44) 20 7368 1654 • Fax: 0(+44) 20 7368 3365 • www.acius.net